MY CRAZY LIFE:
A HUMOROUS GUIDE TO UNDERSTANDING MAST CELL DISORDERS

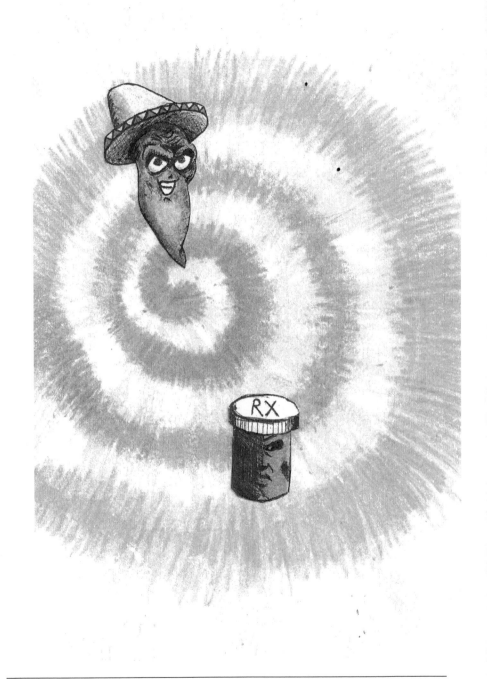

MY CRAZY LIFE:
A HUMOROUS GUIDE TO UNDERSTANDING MAST CELL DISORDERS

Daniel & Pamela Hodge

Cover Illustrated by Bethany Hodge

Daniel & Pamela Hodge
2014

First Printing: 2014

ISBN 978-1-312-51507-9

Daniel Hodge
Indianapolis, IN

Dedications

Pam wants to dedicate this book, *in particular order,* to:

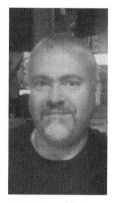

Dan, my loving husband: Thank you for loving me with action when I needed help and for never leaving my side. Thank you for putting this book together for me. Without you, it would not exist.

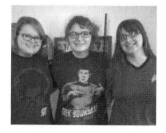

Our children, Gabrielle, Emily, and Bethany: Thank you for enduring all the struggles and altering your life so I can live mine.

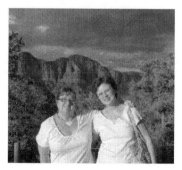

My friend, Connie: Thank you for fulfilling the definition of a friend. Thank you for being there through ups and downs.

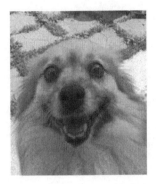 Our dog, Riley: Thank you for sitting outside my bedroom door for months on end. You prove beyond a shadow of doubt that animals love unconditionally and actions speak louder than words.

My broken friendships: I pray that God will give you discernment and you will learn to use it before you speak.

Contents

Foreword

"Sometimes life gives us lessons sent in ridiculous packaging."

Dar Williams

Over the past three years I have learned some valuable lessons. Some lessons didn't cost as much as others. Some lessons I stumbled upon and others I learned the hard way. I have learned that illness can separate and isolate but it can also bring people closer. I have learned that you don't really know someone until you need something from them, then you find out very quickly about their character. I have learned that life is fragile and fleeting and you must handle it with care. You must try to enjoy every moment of every day and recognize that it really is about the small stuff. Here are some of the other lessons I have learned:

Legal Stuff & Introduction

Right off the bat I want to say that I am not a doctor and I don't play one on T.V. I am not writing this to diagnose anyone. It has not been endorsed by the food and drug administration...okay you get the point.

I AM writing this to help identify the bizarre symptoms of Mast Cell Disorders. To help family and friends understand that mast cell disorders can look pretty bizarre. Because of the unpredictable nature of this disease, many people who are close to us tend to jump to the conclusion that we are making up the symptoms or that we are faking. Some will go so far as to say we are crazy or have mental illness.

You would think that getting a diagnosis from a specialist would help curb these accusations. Unfortunately, that is not always the case. I am saddened when I read over and over that someone's mother, wife, friend or husband does not "believe" them, that it is all made up or all in their head. This book is also for you- unbelieving mom, wife, friend and husband.

Imagine, if you will, falling off a bike and breaking your arm. The pain is immediate and real. Now imagine going to the ER and the doctors looking at you and telling you that you are just upset about the accident, nothing is broken. All the while you know it is. You can see the bone sticking out. Now you are told to calm down and sent home. Take a few pills and all will be better. You try to tell your mother, wife, friend or husband that you definably broke your arm. They disagree because the ER doctor said it was fine, it must be fine. A few days go by and your arm is swollen and red, the pain is unbearable. Your mother, wife, friend or husband tells you to get over it, there is no way your arm is broken - it's all in your head.

Now how would you feel? Would you feel loved and cared for? Or would you feel sad and confused about the fact no one can see your broken bone sticking through your skin? Of course you would feel sad and confused. You would have physical pain from the broken arm, but you are also going to have emotional pain from the people so quickly dismissing you as making it up or looking for attention.

Will this ever really happen? No, because modern medicine and technology can x-ray that arm. Anyone with sight can see the bone sticking out. You would get reactions from everyone around you. Someone may even be sick at the sight of the bone sticking out. Someone might feel upset and want to help out, maybe bring you a meal. Someone might even want to sign your cast!

When people can relate to a situation, like a broken arm, they have empathy towards people. They can understand the pain involved and what it will take to heal.

When it comes to rare disorders, very few can have empathy. With a mast cell disorder, things are happening at a cellular level and people can't see that. All they can see is the reactions that occur after a trigger. Their perspective is very one-sided and understandably so. On top of their inability to actually see the mast cells reacting, there are a lot of emotional reactions that people don't understand. Unlike the broken arm, things are physically happening in the body and the brain that cause depression and anxiety, but these things can't always be seen.

Remember, just because you can't see things doesn't mean they are not real. Can you see air? Can you see love?

Can you see gravity? These are things you can't see with the human eye and yet everyone will admit they are real.

X-rays were invented in 1895 by a German physicist named Wilhelm Conrad Röntgen. A little over a hundred years ago people had to use other methods to detect a broken arm. They had to believe what they couldn't see and make educated guesses on how to best go about fixing the problem.

Even with today's modern medicine, mast cells and their functions are a topic of research. Research has barely scratched the surface in diagnosing and treating mast cell disorders. If you consider how rare mast cell disorders are you might understand why your patient-your daughter, husband, friend or wife-seems a bit "odd" or different. It is because they are! They are on the cutting edge of science.

I know I'm odd-I call myself a freak-but in a loving way. I am, like many others, a canary, your canary in a coal mine. What is hurting us is most likely hurting you, but undetected.

From the perspective of my family, all of my reactions are either seen or unseen. They have seen me throw up, but they can't see my throat swell. They have seen me flush and turn red, but they can't see my nausea. There are going to be symptoms that people don't see. At some point you will need to accept that you can't see things on a cellular level but a patient-your daughter, husband, friend or wife-can feel it.

I challenge you to take the time to read this book, to look at the links provided and to do some research into the unknown. Step up instead of stepping back.

I also wrote this to help make the light bulb turn on for patients and to help them connect some dots. In my search for information on Mast Cell Disorders, I never found a book that was not a medical journal intended to be used by a medical student or doctor. So, I am writing this from the patient's perspective.

I AM ONLY AN EXPERT ON MYSELF, NOT OTHERS.

This guide does not list and contain every symptom possible. I do list throughout the guide helpful links and forums that contain extensive lists. Including every list would make this guide into an encyclopedia!

Although Mast Cell Disorders are rare, there is a lot of information about them on the internet. Finding it scattered throughout the internet is the hard part. I have gathered the information for you. I hope to help by having a lot of it in one spot and to help guide you to it.

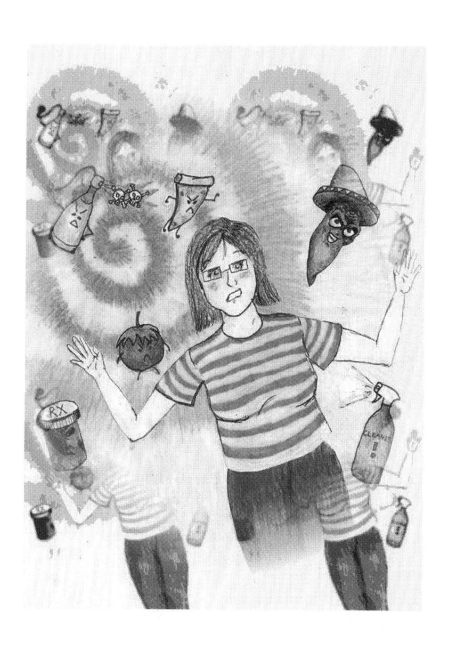

Chapter 1: Mast Cell Disorders

This disorder is not easy to diagnose. In fact, it is one of the last things to look for after years of doctor visits and tests. It is so rare that the patient is often misdiagnosed and therefore not treated with the proper medications.

I think one of the best ways to understand a mast cell disorder is to first understand what a mast cell is and what it does. Mast cells are part of the immune system. Their job is to defend against pathogens and to help heal wounds. They also fight against allergens. They protect us and fight unseen battles going on in the body. When you have a mast cell disorder, you either make too many mast cells or the ones you have start misbehaving, or acting on their own -- firing at will. Too much of a good thing is not always good.

Mast Cell Disorders include Mastocytosis and Mast Cell Activation Syndrome (MCAS). Mast cell disorders can be genetic, but not always. Scientists have found there is a mutation in a gene that causes Mastocytosis. With more research, most likely more genetic markers will be found. There is no cure, but the symptoms of mast cell disorders can be controlled with the proper medication. Mastocytosis can be separated into two categories – Cutaneous Mastocytosis (CM) and Systemic Mastocytosis (SM). CM is considered disease of the skin. The majority of children who have Mastocytosis have the cutaneous form. A large percentage of those children will outgrow it before puberty. People who have Systemic Mastocytosis can have the cutaneous type as well. There are some people who have the cutaneous form and never get the systemic form. You may have heard the saying "Some have spots, some do not", this is referring to having the cutaneous form with spots or the systemic form without spots.

Systemic Mastocytosis comes in several forms. Each of these forms creates havoc in the body and can be life-threatening, some more than others. These include:

Indolent Systemic Mastocytosis (ISM)

Systemic Mastocytosis with associated clonal hematologic non mast cell lineage disease (SM-AHNMD)

Aggressive Systemic Mastocytosis (ASM)-this is a rare form.

Mast Cell Leukemia (MCL)-This form is very rare, the cells are considered malignant or cancerous.

The WHO (World Health Organization) recently started recognizing Mast cell Activation Syndrome (MCAS). A super simplified explanation would be to say with MCAS you have the correct number of mast cells but the ones you have are misbehaving. In fact, they can trigger due to many things, food or smells that are unavoidable throughout one's day or for no reason or cause at all.

With Mastocytosis, for unknown reasons, the body makes too many mast cells and this can cause multiple problems in the skin and organs. Plus you have all those extra mast cells misbehaving.

When misbehaving, the mast cells degranulate or spew histamine, heparin and other chemicals at an alarming rate. This can result in several reactions -- everything from hives, nausea, vomiting, diarrhea, and anaphylaxis.

At this time, treatment is the same for both MCAS and Mastocytosis. So whether you have a mob of mast cells or you have hooligan mast cells, treatment usually starts with H1 and H2 antihistamines. This is usually followed by mast cell stabilizers, if the antihistamines alone are not enough. Mast cell stabilizers include Gastrocrom (generic is call Cromolyn) and Zaditor (generic is called Ketotifen). Ketotifen is not FDA approved in the United States. You can buy the name brand from other countries. It is also legal to get it compounded in the United States. Singulair, a leukotriene inhibitor, has been helpful in treating symptoms as well.

Others have found Xolair to be helpful. Chemotherapy is used for those with mastocytosis if other treatments are not effective.

I am currently taking Allegra (H1) twice a day, Zantac (H2) twice a day, Cromolyn four times a day, and Ketotifen twice a day. Singulair was added last year and has really helped. Strangely, I couldn't tell it was even working until I went off of it. That is when I could tell it had been helping! I started triggering or reacting to many things when I went off of it. So I went right back on it. In case you are wondering, Singulair is a drug for asthma sufferers; however its main job is to block the leukotriene, which is one of the spewing chemicals.

Due to the unpredictable nature of the disease, all mast cell patients should carry two Epi Pens with them at all times unless told otherwise by a doctor. (For patients on Beta Blockers, Glucagon may need to be administered- please discuss this with your doctor). I want to repeat that last sentence...TWO Epi Pens at all times. Originally, I was unaware of the need to carry two all the time. I learned in the ER why you should carry two. I had a rebound anaphylaxis event. I was treated with Epinephrine, steroids, and Benadryl and responded well. For unknown reasons the anaphylaxis returned (rebound) and I had to be treated again. So you always want two doses with you at all times in case the first dose is not enough. Always call for emergency assistance when you need to use an Epi Pen!

What causes the mast cells to misbehave? It is usually triggers or allergens. Although, a true allergy is not needed to have a reaction. To complicate matters, each patient has different triggers that cause degranulation.   Some triggers that cause degranulation are:

-Food

-Medication

-Stress (emotional ups and downs.)

-Scents/Fragrances

-Heat (from the weather or from hot drinks or foods.)

-Cold (again from the weather or from cold drinks or frozen foods.)

-Exercise

-Sex (but who cares, right?)

-Pressure (any kind of pressure - for example, pressure from a CPAP mask, pressure from riding on an airplane, from holding a child, sitting or lying down.)

-Vibration(Including, but not limited to, vibration from riding on an airplane, in a car, bus or train.)

-Mold

-Plants

-Chemicals/Cleaners

-Insect Bites

Mast Cell disorders can be life-changing for the patients and their families. Lifestyles usually have to be altered to keep the patient safe. Symptoms appear at a minute's notice and can be life-threatening. In other words, you can be fine one minute and very ill the next. This, I think, is one of the hardest concepts for family and friends to grasp. We are conditioned to think that serious illness takes weeks or months to occur. This concept goes against the reality of Mast Cell Disorders.

I showed symptoms for years before I got sick. I spent years going to different specialists and getting several diagnoses. I have been diagnosed with everything from Gout, Mixed Connective Tissue Disease, Chronic Fatigue Syndrome and Fibromyalgia. Am I angry about these diagnoses? Na. They were taught to look for horses, not zebras. Do I have these diseases or are they symptoms of the mast cell disorders? Researchers are still trying to figure that out.

When I think of how to explain Mast Cell Disorders as a disease, the first thing I think of is the fact that it does not follow the rules. It is like playing a board game with a cheater, someone who makes the rules up as they go, or changes the rules in their favor. It is always changing and unpredictable. The only certainty is that it is there and you must be vigilant.

There are many symptoms of mast cell disorders. I have put a + sign to indicate my original symptoms before diagnosis.

A list of symptoms include:

skin lesions or sores

skin rash, spots, redness +

hives +

persistent fatigue +

itching

flushing & severe sweating +

joint, bone pain +

persistent diarrhea +

vomiting

hair loss +

mouth sores +

nausea +

swelling & inflammation +

chest pain + (lung pain)

gastrointestinal pain, bloating +

unexplained medication reactions + (I became unable to take most of my medications.)

enlarged liver/spleen

liver/spleen/bladder/kidney pain +

enlarged lymph nodes

frequent urination

recurring infections

neuropathic pain

constipation

unexplained bruising, bleeding

malabsorption

intermittent tinnitus or hearing problems+

odd reactions to insect stings +

anesthesia difficulties

anemia

thyroid problems

decreased bone density

unexplained weakness +

shortness of breath +

sunlight sensitivity +

temperature (hot/cold) sensitivity +

difficulty with foods, drinks + (Salicylates, some dairy and foods high in histamines.)

anaphylactoid reactions +

anaphylaxis +

vision problems

unexplained weight loss (I wish!)

cognitive impairment + (Known as brain fog, some days I have difficulty finding words or completing a sentence.)

sinus problems +

headaches +

tachycardia (racing heart rate)

eyes tearing/dry eyes + (dry eyes for me)

persistent body/tissue pain +

difficulty exercising + (I don't like exercising so this one may not count!)

vertigo

episodes of low body temperature +

Vitamin B12 deficiency

Vitamin D deficiency +

iron deficiency

fragrance/odors/chemical reactions +

difficult menses (females)

numbness & tingling in the extremities and/or face +

skin has a burning sensation

unexplained anxiety +

sudden drops in blood pressure

fainting

flushing +

I also remember feeling total exhaustion.

The symptoms are vast and match symptoms to many other diseases. It is very important when looking at symptoms to know there is a list of other diseases that mimic mast cell diseases, so the other diseases must always be ruled out.

There are also two diseases that have been commonly found in conjunction with mast cell disorders. The first one is Postural Orthostatic Tachycardia syndrome (P.O.T.S) - Symptoms are wide-spread because the autonomic nervous system plays the role of regulating functions in the body. Low blood pressure upon standing, light-headedness and fainting are common symptoms.

The other disease is Ehlers–Danlos syndrome (EDS). It is an inherited connective tissue disorder. There are several types of EDS.

Of the three diseases - mast cell disorders, POTS and EDS, some people have just one and some have a combination of them, while some can have all three.

Here is the link to the list of other diseases to rule out:

http://www.ncbi.nlm.nih.gov/pmc/articles/PMC3069946/table/T4/

Chapter 2: My Journey

"We must be willing to let go of the life we have planned, so as to have the life that is waiting for us."

E.M. Forster

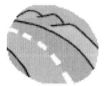 So my journey began about 15 years ago. I believe it started after I had a sinus surgery. I had a horrible head ache and felt very run down. I called every few days to tell them something was not right, and the nurses assured me that what I was feeling was normal. It was not normal. After putting up with these symptoms and calling for a month I broke down in tears and called. I insisted on seeing the doctor, and told them this could not be normal. The doctor accused me of not following the directions and said it looked like I didn't blow my nose. Then he got a good look and said, "Oh, it is packing". I didn't even get a "sorry" from the surgeon... and he didn't get the balance due after our insurance paid! He did get a letter listing the many reasons why it would be better to write off the bill than to send us another one. Before he removed the packing that had adhered to my sinus cavity, he warned me it was going to hurt a little...a little? He also told me it would take another month to heal because removing the packing would make it raw. Recovery was slow. This was, for me, the first sign that something was not quite right. I was bedridden for nearly another month. I never felt the same after this. I had extreme fatigue and strange aches and pains. I had strange symptoms off and on.

Over the next 15 years my symptoms increased. I saw many specialists, including a rheumatologist, an endocrinologist, and a dermatologist. I even went to an alternative allergist and massage therapists. I was searching for someone to help me feel better.

When my youngest started school I went back to work. So feeling tired all the time was normal, I thought. I did find out that I had sleep apnea, which I am sure contributed to the tiredness.

The rheumatologist found that my ANAs or antinuclear antibodies were high, 1:160. This is a sign that the body is fighting itself. The ANA pattern was speckled. Because of this pattern and the fact that other tests did not show anything unusual, the rheumatologist diagnosed me with Fibromyalgia. My vitamin D level was also extremely low.

Looking back over the years, I can see little signs of mast cell issues. One year I was stung by a sweat bee. A teeny tiny sweat bee caused my leg to get infected and to swell. I had to take steroids to get it under control. On top of that, I was nursing my baby and was told I couldn't nurse her for 10 days. I had to pump for 10 days while the baby screamed. This is the week we found out that she was lactose intolerant! I'm not sure who was more thrilled when those 10 days were up-the baby or me!

I have also had extremely strange reactions to certain drugs. My strangest reaction was to sulfa drugs.

More recently I developed a bad case of bronchitis and that is when things went downhill! I was accurately treated with antibiotics and steroids. The bronchitis went away, but the joint pain that I had for years increased. I was exhausted. I would come home from work and go straight to bed. Anyone who knows me knows I love to cook and eat. So for me to skip a meal meant something was not right. I noticed that my skin was constantly flushing, my hair started falling out, my nails became like paper and they would just tear off. I noticed that the fluorescent lighting made my flesh feel like it was on fire! At work I would wear long sleeves every day and hats on occasion so my scalp wasn't being burnt.

Though my symptoms were progressing, the rheumatologist did not want to change his diagnosis. So I found a new rheumatologist. My ANA's continued to rise even higher. They were 1:320. The doctor said she thought it looked like Lupus, and prescribed Hydroxychloroquine (Plaquenil). I just figured it had been lurking in the background for some time. Though you hate to be diagnosed with horrible things, at least you know what's going on. She did a SED rate test. A few weeks later when the test came back she said the SED rate was not elevated enough for Lupus. She said perhaps it was Mixed Connective Tissue Disease. I needed to stay on the current treatment because Plaquenil would help with that, as well. I developed more symptoms: I started to get kidney pain and lung pain. The doctor and I both thought the lung pain was Pleurisy, but this is something that goes along with Lupus, and I didn't have Lupus. Thankfully, she treated me with steroids and that helped with the pain. However, it came and went for months.

I never ever ask if things can get worse, because they certainly can.

One Sunday my husband and I enjoyed a dinner theater after church. The food was a buffet; usually roast beef, chicken, veggies, fruit and a wonderful salad bar. Because we had eaten such a large lunch, we just had a little scoop of ice cream instead of dinner. I would call it the dessert I didn't have earlier! A few hours later, around bed time, I noticed that my throat felt a little funny... It was thick, or full. It was uncomfortable, but not unbearable. It felt like it needed to be cleared. So I started looking on the internet for possible reasons. (Doctors don't really like this.) I saw that an enlarged thyroid could be causing it. I had a hard time sleeping that night because of the constant discomfort of needing to clear my throat. You know -- one of those nights where you watch the clock as it gets closer to the time the alarm is set to go off. It was a long night and I was supposed to work the next day, but I was feeling like work was the last thing I could do. So I called around and found someone to take my shift. That was the first day of work that I had missed. Even through the Lupus diagnosis, then the Mixed Connective Tissue diagnosis, I had not missed a day of work. After a day or so my throat went back to normal.

Later that week, I developed a strange looking brownish-red rash on my leg. It wasn't itchy, and it was under the skin; very odd. It looked more like spots!

After a few days, it looked almost like I had developed a different rash in the same location. The new rash was itchy and broke the skin. It started out small and grew. I called the doctor and they told me to stop the Plaquenil, I was probably having an allergic reaction to it. Great! So I stopped it, but the rash continued to grow and by that evening, my throat started having that funny feeling again. This time I knew that it was an allergic reaction, not an enlarged thyroid. When I realize that the throat situation was getting worse, not better, I woke up my husband and told him I thought I needed to go to the hospital. It was frightening; it took extra effort to move air and swallow.

At the ER they administered epinephrine, Benadryl and steroids. I told them about the Plaquenil and how I was told to stop it. They took me down for a CAT scan of my throat. I'm not sure why, maybe to make sure that I didn't have that enlarged thyroid after all! On the way there, I started vomiting. What a mess. After getting back to the ER room and resting a while, I started to rebound. It was like the epinephrine had worn off and it all started over. They came in and gave me more of the same. That is when they explained the rebound effect. (Repeating: If you have a prescription for an EpiPen, this is why you should carry two with you at all times). I had no idea this could happen. It was the strangest thing. I was so much better after the first dose of epinephrine, Benadryl and steroids, and then *boom*, out of nowhere, it all started over. I'm telling you, that is some scary stuff! I was given a prescription for steroids for the rash that had grown from my knee up my torso. They agreed that I was having an allergic reaction to the Plaquenil and I was released after being monitored for several hours.

I want to make an important point here for women. I was having my period at the time of this reaction. Hormones can affect your mast cells. They can make you very sensitive and cause you to react. I have found this to be true time and time again. For this reason I pretty much stay home for those days out of the month. It is better to be safe than to be in the ER!

I know now that this was my first of many anaphylactic reactions. I was on the steroid for 10 days. As soon as the steroid wore off, the rash reappeared as well as the anaphylaxis. So I ended up back in the ER. I was sent home with steroids again, only for it to continue to happen. I got in to see the rheumatologist, and she had no choice but to do another round of the steroids. In the meantime, the kidney and lung pain was ridiculous. I went to visit my regular doctor and he did a urine test and chest X-rays. The X-rays came out fine. The urine test came back positive for blood, but negative for infection, which he thought was a kidney stone. He called for a CAT scan of my kidneys, but could not find the stone. I now think that I was suffering from IC (Interstitial cystitis). IC can be caused by mast cells and affects the bladder and sometimes the kidneys. You can read more about IC here:

http://mastcellmaster.com/documents/Interstitial-Cystitis/Mast-cells-IC-Urol-2007.pdf

I think I was glowing from all the scanning going on. A few weeks later, I was back in the office with lung pain so bad I couldn't help but sit in the waiting room and cry. The doctor ordered another lung x-ray. Nothing showed up. Now I was ticked off. I didn't understand how something could hurt so badly and not show up. In fact, I still don't get that!

Again, never ever ask if things can get worse.

My husband and I went to our friend's wedding. The wedding cake was delicious. It was cheesecake. Yum! They also served finger foods, cute little sandwiches, veggies, and fruits. It was a lovely time and I'm glad they included us in their celebration. We had a great time. Unfortunately, my throat started swelling on the way home. That was terrifying. We had no idea where a hospital was, so we took the first exit and looked for a store. We finally found one, ran in, and ripped the box of Benadryl open in the middle of the aisle. I took two and tried to calm down. I was afraid to leave the store because that meant getting back on the unfamiliar highway. I think about how lucky I was that I didn't have a rebound reaction on the highway! The thought of that still frightens me. Maybe we should have called 911 then. I don't know.

What I do know is that nothing has been the same since that day! I have been told that I am not the fun Pam any longer. Maybe this is the day that I changed. I used to love adventure, but now I want to stay close to home, close to the familiar where I can control the environment. It had been several weeks since the rash incident and taking the Plaquenil, so I couldn't figure out why I was having this happen all over again.

So this episode spurred me to see an allergist/immunologist. He prescribed Epi Pens on my first visit. Obviously, he knew something I didn't. I figured "Okay, that would be good just in case it ever does happen again".

He did extensive allergy testing and found out that I was allergic to...Nothing! No IGE allergies. This is another important note, remember this!

Next, I had some chemical patch testing done. This is to look for contact allergies of the skin. With this they found that I did have 6 or 7 chemical allergies, which is considered a lot. Most are chemicals found around me at any given time: cement, epoxy, fragrance, nickel, and Mercapto Mix. Mercapto mix is found in shoes, adhesives, electrical plugs and cords, mats, headphones, gloves, condoms, rubber bands, neoprene and medical tubing like the kind I use with my C-Pap machine. Obviously, total avoidance is impossible.

I started waking up with swollen lips and eyes and I started having diarrhea on a daily basis. My husband and I noticed a pattern. The morning after a romantic encounter, I would be puffy in the eyes and lips. It seriously looked like things got a little rough! I can assure you they did not, but to look at me you would certainly wonder. We brought that to the attention of the allergist. He informed us that it is possible for women to be allergic to their spouse's semen. He thought that I had become allergic to my husband. You have to wonder how this is even possible. We had been married for 17 years. Now, out of the blue, I was allergic to him? This did not make any sense. To this day I am still trying to wrap my head around this one. This crazy disease has done a lot to make my life rough, but now it was affecting my husband on a personal level, as well.

The allergist informed us that we could be treated for this, or we could just use condoms. If we were to be treated, it would have to be in a hospital. We have three children and are not looking to have any more, so we chose the latter option. This sounds like an easy fix, but then we had to find a condom that I didn't react to. It just keeps getting more and more complicated.

My stomach had been hurting for several months. It felt as if someone had just punched me. The allergist sent me to see a gastroenterologist to have an upper GI with biopsies done on my stomach. The gastroenterologist suggested that I also have a colonoscopy. However, the prep for the colonoscopy caused my throat to swell. So I wasn't able to have that procedure done. The good news was that my stomach looked okay, but I had some reflux issues that needed to be dealt with. Also, according the biopsy, I was negative for celiac. However, at the time of the biopsy the doctors were not looking for mast cells, so unfortunately no slides were taken to look for extra mast cells in the stomach.

I know now that the just-punched-in-the-stomach feeling I had was probably my mast cells degranulating, or opening up. I also believe my gut was sick. My stomach felt like it was a mess. There is another feeling that I think comes from the mast cells degranulating. It's a feeling I can only describe as your insides moving, shaking or squirming. I call it purring, because to me it feels like I'm purring. This is an odd feeling, but doesn't particularly hurt. I feel this mostly in the early mornings. It will sometimes wake me. I am guessing this is because histamines naturally peak in the early morning. If I have an abundance of histamines, I will have a fast heart beat and have a hard time sleeping. Insomnia is a common symptom with mast cell disorders.

My specialist recently had my ANA's retested and they were elevated even higher at 1:1280. This is very high. My specialist referred me to yet another Rheumatologist, one she knows personally. He ran $2000 worth of tests. The conclusion was that the mast cells are causing my problems. Right now he does not think I have lupus. He said if I wake up with a butterfly rash someday it will be an easy diagnosis. I asked him if the mast cell reactions were causing the high ANAs or if the high ANAs were causing the mast cell reaction. His answer -- YES! They just don't know enough about mast cell disease yet to be sure.

Chapter 3: Home

"When I speak of home, I speak of the place where those I love are gathered together; and if that place were a gypsy's tent, or a barn, I should call it by the same good name notwithstanding."

Charles Dickens

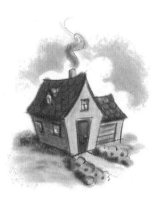

I love this quote by Charles Dickens; I painted it on the riser of my stairway several years ago. Little did I know at the time what this quote would be foretelling.

The bad became worse when I started going into anaphylaxis randomly... at least I thought it was random. One of the hardest days was the day that I could not stand to be in my house. I walked into the house and my throat started to swell and I broke out in hives. I ran out the front door, waited a few minutes and tried it again, with no success, I might add. What do you do? What could I do? My whole world was being turned upside down and I couldn't even go into my home. Making matters worse, I had to work the next day!

I begged my youngest daughter Bethany to stay with me in the SUV. She was 16 and camping in the car with mom was not one of her favorite things to do. I knew this, but I was afraid to be alone. I was afraid of what was happening. I couldn't ask my husband because he needed to get a good night's sleep because he is up and off for work very early every morning. So, Bethany was a trooper. We stayed in the SUV for two nights and I could do it no longer, however, I still could not go into the house. Left with very few options we went and bought a tent and did some real camping in the back yard! Unfortunately, it was in the heat of the summer and we were miserable in the tent.

I continued to work. My husband would gather my clothes and we would go to the Y for me to shower. Thankfully, we were members. There is a medical building next to our house and I went there to use the bathroom. I now understand why homeless people don't look their best. It is hard to live outside and look good!

Of course, I called the doctor and I went in. He added another medicine to my antihistamines.

After a week in the tent, I begged my husband to put us in a motel. I am not a great camper after all. After moving into a motel, I thought I was living the life! I had a shower and a bed!

Amazing how fast life can change your perspectives.

During all of this, I had to leave work early one day and go to the immediate care center. I was being treated by a very nice Nurse Practitioner. She told me that something in my home was probably to blame for all of this and I should try to find it. Very good advice! So we hired mold inspectors to analyze the house. They said the carbon dioxide level was too high, which indicated mold. But the mold levels were acceptable. Another important note I want to add here: it is important to hire a mold inspector, NOT a mold remediator to do the inspection. You want a company that will not benefit from finding mold in your house. You can later hire a mold remediation company if you find a mold problem.

I was so physically tired and mentally drained. I know my husband was terribly stressed as well (along with the checkbook). After a week in the motel we traveled 45 minutes north to stay with my mother-in-law. She was nice enough to take us in! My middle daughter, Emily, who was 19, stayed in the house. She was working and going to school. We stayed a week with my mother-in-law. It was a stressful week. Between driving back and forth to work, I was having anaphylaxis every few days and my mother-in-law thought I was over-reacting to the whole situation. I really don't know how you can over-react to the fact that you are allergic to your husband, your house and your favorite foods, but, regardless, everyone has an opinion. I believe she was mourning the loss of her husband and we may have stressed her. So we resided at a motel once again. As the days turned into weeks, I became a bit more frazzled you could say. I was working, dealing with my mystery illness and living out of a suitcase in a motel. At least my husband was with me. Bethany would go from the motel to home, stay a few days here and a few days there. Nothing like stability for a teenager!

As funds ran low, we devised a plan to partition a room off in the house. My husband went to the home improvement store and purchased a roll of thick plastic and duct tape. On the government website they give instructions on how to handle a biological emergency. To us, this was an emergency. So we moved all the furniture out of the dining room into the living room. We had dining room and living room furniture stacked to the ceiling. We put plastic all around making a plastic bubble for me to stay in. Instead of the Boy In The Plastic Bubble, it was The Middle Aged Woman In The Plastic Bubble. Not an Academy Award winner! I was able to stay in the bubble room. It turned out to be a good option for a few days, but I still felt ill. I found that if I wore a mask I could go out of the plastic bubble.

Thankfully, I had some great friends who offered me a spare bed. This gave me respite, so to speak, from the house. Thanks Karen, Connie, and Sara!

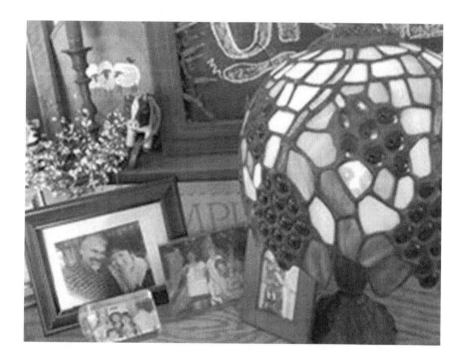

Chapter 4: Miracles

"There are only two ways to live your life. One is as though nothing is a miracle. The other is as though everything is a miracle."

Albert Einstein

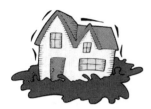 One day we noticed water coming out from under the wall. OH MY GOODNESS! At this point I felt like I was being punished. How many other things could go wrong? Water was just rushing out from under the wall into the family room, laundry room and garage. One would think that water would originate in the laundry room, but no. Water was coming out of the wall. So we started cleaning that mess up. While mopping the small pond I remembered that a few years back the same thing had happened, but only once. I began to wonder if this happened before perhaps that is where the mold is. It could be in the wall that is spewing the water! So we did what any stressed out crazy people would do. We went to the garage side of the wall and started taking down the drywall. I did switch to an N95 mask for extra protection from the mold we were going to find. Now, my wonderful husband is an accountant, not a man of construction, but he did a fabulous job taking down that wall. He was my hero! He says "*De*struction is easy; it's *con*struction that is hard, even as a general rule of life." He is a smart man.

We were finally going to find the nasty stuff and all because we had this horrible flood in the family room. These dreams were short-lived. We had the wall completely taken down. There we found...nothing, nada, no mold anywhere. The wall was relatively dry. The insulation was dry. But the bottom of the wall was wet. The framing was wet at the bottom. We had given it our best and it wasn't good enough, so we called out the troops. We had construction workers, roofers, and even a plumber come and look at the problem. None of them could figure it out either. The water had stopped flowing as fast as it had started. Now there was no water and no mold. This was a real mystery, a real unsolved mystery.

A week or so later the water started flowing from the wall again. I was livid. My husband, being the calm, level person was also upset, but not as much as I was. I wanted to rip that area completely out. There was a ceiling and an adjacent wall. Maybe the water was coming from there. I felt like the hulk. You know, right when he turns green and goes a little crazy. Except I didn't rip my clothes off, I just ripped the ceiling off! Wearing my N95 mask and with anger surging through me, being frustrated from months of turmoil. With tears and anger I was taking it all out on the wall. I tore down the ceiling and the adjacent wall. I don't think I could have been stopped. Any married man out there knows there are times in a relationship where it is best just to step back and let the poo poo hit the fan. This was that time. Dan knew to step aside or he might get hurt, too. I just used my hands and tore the living day lights out of that area. When I was done it was a heaping mess of drywall and dust. I had made a terrible mess.

My little anger fit had revealed the duct work to the furnace, but no sign of a leak or mold. However with a step latter you could see the entire length of the dropped ceiling in the laundry room. Wouldn't it be nice if a builder would leave a copy of the blue prints with every house built? That would help identify where all the ducts went. We had the whole place torn apart, so we inspected it closely. With flashlights we looked at each duct and each connection. Some of the connections were covered with insulation. At this point we have to buy new insulation anyway, so we started taking the old stuff down. That was the smartest thing we could have done, because that is when we found it! It was there the whole time, but not at all related to the mysterious leaking wall. There it was in all its nastiness, mold covering the insulation that was wrapped around the duct. Two pieces of the duct work were pulled apart and the condensation from the heat and the air conditioning had created ideal conditions for mold. Because of its location, every time the heat or air kicked on, the mold was being thrown all over the house. We had the furnace repair man come out to repair the duct work. He said that it appeared that it was never installed and connected correctly when the house was built. You have to wonder why someone would do their job half way and then cover it up with insulation.

Now the real clean-up must begin. We got rid of all the furniture that could hold the mold spores, anything cloth. I thought perhaps I was allergic to the mold spores. I have a good friend, Karen, who came over and helped me do the hard work of deciding what to get rid of. If it couldn't be washed in bleach water, it pretty much had to go. We washed every surface in the house with bleach water, in hopes of killing all the mold spores. We also ran air cleaners 24/7. The hope was that I could stay in the house and get out of the bubble room at the expense of getting rid of most of the furniture and decorations.

We rotated between motels and the bubble room. Back at home, the water stopped leaking once again. A few days later it started flowing again. Remembering that I had recently turned on the air conditioner, we realized that the air conditioner may have been the problem all along. We called the repairman again. It turns out the drain line on the air conditioner was clogged.

I was also having trouble going to church. At first, I thought it was all the fragrances, but it became obvious later that there was more to it. For hours after church, my lungs would burn and that is not the symptom that exposure to fragrance causes me. We were told later that the church had some water/flooding issues. So, essentially, I became the human mold detector. I still have that skill to this day! There are a couple of buildings I cannot go into and have assumed it is due to hidden mold. I recently found out that both buildings have had water problems in the past.

If it wasn't for the water flowing out of the wall, we would have never looked there for the mold. I originally thought the water was a punishment, now I think it was a miracle!

Chapter 5: Travels

"Where we love is home-home that our feet may leave but not our hearts."

Oliver Wendell Holmes

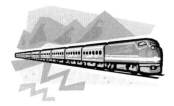 My health really wasn't improving on a regimen of antihistamines and living in the bubble. We assumed it was from the mold exposure in the house and maybe the library building. So my husband and I decided it would be best if I left the house for an extended period of time. This would also give him a much needed break from my never-ending lists of problems. So, I took Bethany, my little camping buddy, and we headed out west. We took Amtrak to Arizona where my parents live. This is a two day trip one way. I was nervous about getting on a train for two days, but I had my EpiPens and enough Benadryl to tranquilize a horse!

Once there, my symptoms did improve some but I still went into anaphylaxis occasionally. I had a nice visit with my parents; however August is not the best month to visit southern Arizona. It is not only a dry heat, it is a 118 degree heat--that is too hot, no matter what kind of heat it is! We stayed shy of a month. While we were in Arizona, Dan emptied out the mini-barn, just in case I still couldn't stay in the house when I got home. What a job for him. We have lived in the house many years and the barn proved it. It was full of bikes, skates and softball bats from the kids' childhood. We stored all of our Christmas Decoration there along with all the tools and lawn care items. He took all the items from the barn and moved them to the garage. That in itself is a huge job, but then he noticed the window of the barn was rotting. Now one job turned into two jobs. The window would need replaced and the rotting wood removed. Thankfully our pastor was willing to help with this repair. He is a crafty man and had all the knowledge and tools needed for the job. This, however, was not the relaxing time I was hoping Dan would have.

This was also the week that the insurance adjuster came for a visit. She came out to inspect the flood damages. What she found was probably shocking and amusing. She found the family room in total disarray from moving all the furniture to one side of the room to get it away from the flood waters. Further in the house she found a bubble room and a living room stacked to the ceiling with dining room furniture. On further inspection the garage was impassable due to the items from the mini barn.

I can only imagine what went through her head. I am glad I was not here to witness it! This was a perfect snapshot of our lives. The chaos was evident.

Later we got a letter from the insurance company stating they were concerned that we were hoarders and we had six months to get the house cleaned up or they were going to drop us. They did come out six months later and took photos. They wanted proof!

It really is too bad that she didn't see the mini-barn -- it looked great!

Chapter 6: Chalet

"Home is any four walls that enclose the right person."

Helen Rowland

The two-day trip home was filled with excitement. I had a wonderful visit with my parents, but the trip was long and I was ready to be home. I was sure that the house would be clean enough. Dan had kept the windows open most of the time to air out any remaining mold spores. He put fans in the window to draw everything outside.

Dan picked us up at the train station at midnight. He had reserved a motel for the night. It was late and we were all too tired to deal with the house.

The next morning the moment of truth came...with excitement I walked up to the front door. Behind this door was my old life... I wanted it back so badly. I had spent 3 months sleeping in an SUV, a tent, and motels. I had moved from house to house of friends and relatives. I was exhausted from living in different places. I just wanted to be home, in my home.

We walked in, but within minutes it was obvious that I was not going to be able to stay in the house. How can this be? There is nothing left to clean, nothing left to do, short of getting rid of everything we own. I was exhausted and devastated.

That evening my husband and kids went to a family reunion. I was too tired, disappointed and barely hanging on to my sanity. I didn't go to the reunion. Instead, I spent the evening crying in the mini barn on a blow up mattress that kept losing air. I was crushed and was convinced we needed to sell the house.

There was no place left to go. There was no more money for motels. We looked into a few rentals, but the cost of those exceeded our budget. So the next day we went out and bought flooring and a new bed. It took us an entire day to insulate the mini barn. We didn't do any fancy drywall just plastic over the insulation. We laid down a large sheet of linoleum. It was pretty. It had a wood grain pattern. It looked cozy and warm. Like a log cabin. The new bed came next. By the time we finished the floor it was starting to rain and getting dark, as if the day wasn't depressing enough. We called some friends with a big truck to help us carry the bed home. Thankfully he was available and willing to help us. He hauled it home for us and helped us set it up. Thanks, Michael. I'm not sure you know how much we appreciated your help in this very trying time.

Dan and I moved into the mini-barn that evening. Yes, our mini-barn. Never say never. Life can turn on a dime and sometimes you have to do some crazy things to get by. This was totally against the HOA rules, but we were out of choices. We called it the "Chalet" and made the best of a bad situation. I always have thought it would be really cool to convert an old barn into a house. This was on a much smaller scale – 12 x 16. We had room for a full size bed, dresser, end table and, of course, a t.v. We hung a little curtain up in the corner and purchased a camping toilet for late night potty breaks. If I was really sick I would avoid the house and use the bathroom next door at the medical building. As I mentioned before, I would shower at the Y.

We spent many cool fall evenings snuggled in the bed watching TV. There really wasn't any place else to sit and the lighting wasn't great for reading. I look back now and think this must have made us stronger as a couple. Not too many distractions in a mini-barn!

I eventually hung some quilts up to cover the ugly plastic. I used a staple gun to hang them...it was a barn after all. They were a nice addition to a dreary situation and they seemed to brighten the place up.

Since it was in the fall and getting very cold at night, we used a portable heater, which made me nervous. You hear about those causing fires and our mini barn only had one exit.

I am not sure how many people in the neighborhood figured out we were living in the barn. Our house is in the front of the neighborhood so there are always cars driving by. I'm betting people were thinking "they must be really working hard on a project in that barn; they are always walking out there." It probably became a bit more interesting to see us walking into the house in our PJ's. Our next door neighbor did stop me one day and asked "Pam, are you living in your barn?" I replied "um...yes". Then I went through the story of how I STILL couldn't stay in my house. She offered me a room and a shower. Thanks, Melinda! I appreciated that, but I was tired of moving around and as bad as it sounds to live in a mini-barn, at least I was at home with my husband and the kids were in the vicinity.

Our plan at this point was just to sell the house. We had it inspected by a mold specialist. The house showed the normal amount of mold. We were informed that all houses have mold, I was just hypersensitive. When we actually looked into selling the house, we were told the timing was awful; it was just after the housing bubble bust. If we sold the house, we would lose twenty to thirty thousand dollars! My heart sank. Dan was also concerned that a new house would have similar issues. We were between a rock and a hard spot.

When I think back now to the Chalet, I have a warm, cozy, fuzzy feeling. This was probably one of the hardest months of our married life. At the time, I know I wasn't feeling warm and fuzzy. Now I can clearly see the effort our friends put into helping us and I can see the love my husband had for me to stay with me in that barn.

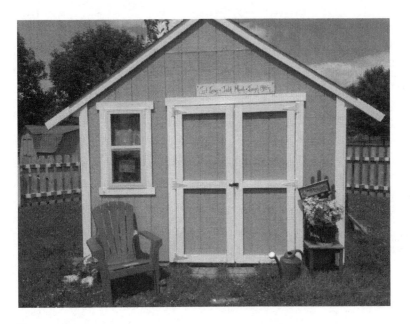

The Chalet.

"Deep into that darkness peering, long I stood there, wondering, fearing, doubting, dreaming dreams no mortal ever dared to dream before."

Edgar Allan Poe

My symptoms waxed a waned between diarrhea, hives, mouth sores, low grade fever, strange bruising and anaphylaxis. I was a mess. I was seeing the doctor monthly with no improvement on my medicine regimen. He tested me for everything under the sun. It all came back negative. He told me about Carcinoid Syndrome. It is uncommon. It is a cancerous tumor hidden somewhere in your body. It presents itself like an allergic reaction. The most obvious symptom is flushing. I fit that to description to a T. At the same time the specialist asked if I had heard of Mastocytosis. He wrote it down on a piece of paper and told me to look it up on the internet. I did and I fit that description, as well. At the time I was still red as a beet, my lungs and my kidneys were still hurting, and I kept going into anaphylaxis. I fit the descriptions of both diseases. So I was being tested for a hidden cancerous tumor or a rare disorder that sounded equally bad. As you can imagine I was feeling a bit low.

The doctor prescribed another round of blood work. I was starting to know the girls at the lab on a first name basis! Sue, one of the women there has always been so nice to me. Even when I looked horrible and was frazzled beyond belief, she always treated me kindly. It is those acts of kindness that make a huge difference to people who are ill. She did for me what she could--she treated me like a friend. She reminds me a lot of my very good friend Lori C., who moved away several years ago and I miss dearly.

I really respect my doctor, but I'm tired, hurting, and living in a mini-barn! I know now that my allergist was systematically ruling everything else out. At the time I just thought he was dragging his feet and felt he wasn't really caring about me. I decided while waiting on test results I would take the results I had and see a new allergist in a different city. My husband took off work to go with me to this appointment. When we got there, I noticed several awards hanging on the wall. I felt deep down that I had come to the right decision to get a second opinion. I had visions of this doctor looking at the records and saying "oh yes, this is what it is". I thought a fresh set of eyes could connect the dots. For a moment I was convinced that we were close to the answers, that this new doctor was going to give me hope, and I would be better in no time at all!

That is not exactly how the visit went.

The doctor looked at my records; spoke with me, asked me some questions. He specifically asked me about my specialist. He told me he knew him and that he was a good doctor and then... he refused me as a patient. I didn't even know doctors did this! The guy did not want to deal with me and all of my mysterious issues. I was devastated once again. At this point all that was missing was the blow up mattress that kept losing air. I felt crushed all over again. I'm glad that my husband was with me and was driving, because I cried all the way home. I wouldn't have been able to see the road to get home. I was thinking at this point, there was no hope of figuring this out.

So it was back to the Chalet. My dreams of a miracle fix and moving back into the house were over. My sweet husband lived with me in the mini-barn 16 days...It felt like

16 weeks. On the morning of the last day, I woke up to horrible exhaust fumes. My breathing was labored and I thought there is no way this could be better than the house. My husband came home on his lunch break and we moved the new bed into our bedroom. He went that day and bought the mother of all air cleaners. It stands 3 feet high and has a HEPA filter, a Hyper-HEPA filter and a charcoal filter. That day we made my "Clean room". We shut off all heating and cooling registers and covered them with plastic. We removed any item that didn't need to be in there. I resided in my clean room from September 2011 to October 2013. Yes, that is two long years in one room. To be fair, it is a large bedroom, like a small studio apartment. If I did go into other parts of the house, I would wear a medical mask. I continued to react to the rest of the house, the trouble was lessened due to the drugs I was taking but I could still feel something affecting me.

In my room of solitude, I had a microwave, a mini fridge and a little electric skillet that I used to cook my food. Thankfully, my family would come and visit me. We would watch movies and sometimes eat dinner together! Cleaning the rest of the house was up to those who were living there, two teenage daughters and my husband. I am guessing that it looked like a fraternity house most of the time. That's okay. I couldn't see it!

Here is the link to the super duper awesome air cleaner:

http://www.iqair.com/

Note: Himalayan Salt lamps are a natural way to help clean the air, along with house plants. These will not replace a good air cleaner, but will assist in keeping the air clean.

The following is a chart of NASA's study on plants that clean the air. It tells you what plants are best and what chemical they remove from the air.

http://en.wikipedia.org/wiki/NASA_Clean_Air_Study

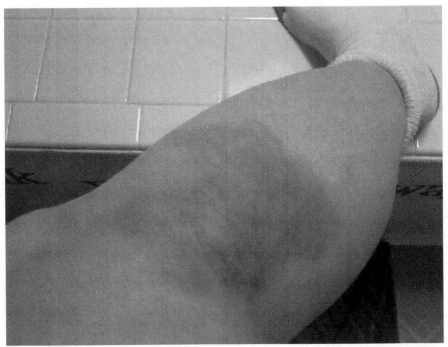

Strange large bruise from a hula hoop.

Chapter 8: Broken Health

"When you are young and healthy, it never occurs to you that in a single second your whole life could change."

Annette Funicelle

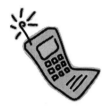 One afternoon I got "the" phone call. The doctor's nurse called and said that the test results were back and I needed to come in and discuss them with the doctor. Of course I wasn't going to let the conversation end like that. I started asking questions and got some vague answers. She said my tryptase was not normal. I asked what that meant, and she said it would be best to talk it over with the doctor. I made an appointment. It took me a couple of weeks to get in to see him, so if it was something really bad they would have had me come in sooner, right?

After waiting on pins and needles for that appointment, the day had finally come! I was having anaphylaxis daily and was in a fight or flight mode most of the time. If I wasn't in the fight or flight mode, I was asleep. I now know it can take up to a week to recover from an episode of anaphylaxis. I was sleeping a lot. I was also taking some very heavy duty antihistamines including, Atarax. Atarax is a strong antihistamine as well as a medicine that is sedating; it helps with the fight or flight, freaking out thing!

Thankfully, my Carcinoid test came back negative! By ruling out Carcinoid, the arrows pointed to Mastocytosis. The doctor told me that I would need to get a Bone Marrow Biopsy (BMB) to confirm the Mastocytosis. At the same time he told me there are lots of false negatives with BMBs. The needle has to go into the exact spot in the bone where the extra mast cells are. I have read some people have had to suffer through up to six BMBs before they could positively diagnose Mastocytosis. That is a lot of drilling! I have the order to get the BMB done, but at this time treatment with the mast cell stabilizer is working and I am more stable. The doctor has allowed me to wait on this procedure, and let me decide when I want it done. I have the understanding that this could change at any time and I am okay with that. Sometimes a BMB will need to be done right away in case you need aggressive treatment. Each case is individual. Find a good specialist and follow their lead.

If you fit the criteria of Mastocytosis and have a BMB but it comes out negative, you likely will fall under the MCAS diagnosis or perhaps it was a false negative. The tests for MCAS are not completely reliable at this time, but a good specialist can diagnose you based on your symptoms, ruling everything else out and your response to mast cell stabilizers.

My doctor told me that I was allergic to the world. Basically, my body was over-reacting—to everything. When he told me this, I don't think I was upset as much as relieved. Relieved that he got it, that he understood why I lived in a bubble room and a mini-barn. He understood and believed me. It is a great feeling when the doctor believes you! Thank heavens someone knew what was going on. I really don't know how much longer I could have gone on. Physically and emotionally I was at my breaking point.

Here is one of the best resources available for you and your doctor.

http://www.tmsforacure.org/documents/Chroni-clesSE.pdf

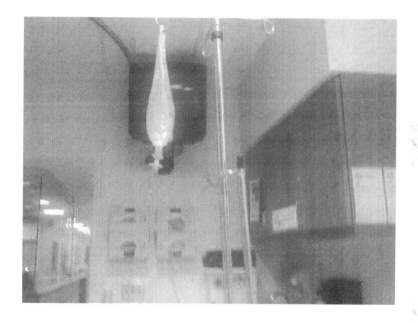

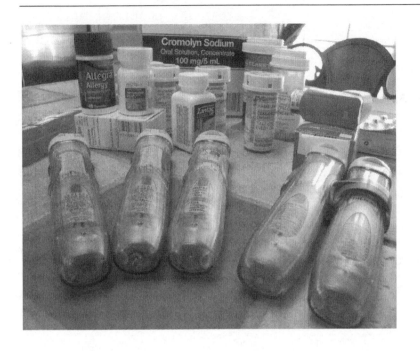

Chapter 9: My Experience With Mast Cell Stabilizers

"The only source of knowledge is experience."

Albert Einstein

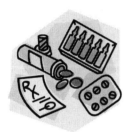 So treatment began! I was put on mast cell stabilizers. The first one I was prescribed was Ketotifen. It is not FDA approved in the United States. Not being FDA approved means it's a little harder to get ahold of and your insurance may not pay for it. You can get Ketotifen from other countries or through compounding pharmacies here in the US. When I first started the Ketotifen, I was extremely sleepy. I have read that people will start Ketotifen on the weekend so that they can just sleep the entire week end. Since my kids are gown and I can't work, anyway, I basically just slept a few weeks.

Slowly I saw improvements in what I could eat. At the time I was only able to eat about 5 foods: beef, chicken, eggs, potatoes and green beans. By this point I had discovered that I have a salicylate sensitivity. Salicylate are in many, many foods and can cause serious reactions in people who are sensitive to them.

Ketotifen was an amazing medicine because it enabled me to eat! I was hungry and the medicine tends to increase your appetite. Between the medicine making me hungry and the fact I could actually eat food, I gain some weight. This is a benefit to people who are under weight. This is one benefit that I certainly did not need! Nevertheless, I was happy!

A month or two later I was put on Cromolyn Sodium, which is generic for Gastrocrom. This is the only FDA approved treatment for Mastocytosis in the US.

When taking Cromolyn Sodium, you must start slowly and work your way up to a full dose. It is the hardest medicine I have ever started. It makes you feel pretty bad. It kind of exacerbated my symptoms. I remember trying to go to the store and having my normal symptoms. I started crying in the parking lot. I thought that this was supposed to help me not hurt me. I felt like I was even more sensitive than before and I had a really horrible headache that lasted a few weeks. I was extremely disappointed, but I hung in there. The sensitivity diminished and the headache went away! You just have to give it time to work. It does NOT work like pain medicine...it is NOT immediate. In fact, it is very slow working, but it does work!

I have read that many people just stop taking it. I felt like I had no choice. I could not live with my untreated symptoms. Now, I'm not telling you this to scare anyone out of taking Cromolyn, just the opposite. I believe Cromolyn saved my life. It took eight days to feel improvement, but improvement did come! Slowly, I regained my strength. I remember on the eighth day I got out of bed and took the dog on a walk. It was a short walk. I had not done that in months. I went into the kitchen and baked muffins. There was a glimpse of the old me shining through!

When people have asked what to expect from starting Cromolyn, I tell them it is like pouring water into a fish tank. You have a nice clear fish tank with fish swimming around. Then you pour a gallon of water in, and you stir everything up. It is so cloudy you can hardly see the fish. You have fish poo and fish food and all kinds of stuff just floating everywhere. That's what starting Cromolyn is like. It stirs everything up and only time can settle everything down. When it does settle down, it is much better than before you started it.

I have read that it can take up to four months for Cromolyn to reach full effectiveness. I think it took me almost six months to feel stable.

For me, Cromolyn has been a wonder drug! It helped with a lot of bone pain and pain that I think was considered fibromyalgia pain. I know they are doing drug studies with fibromyalgia patients and Ketotifen, the other mast cell stabilizer. It sounds like they may be onto something there! Before I was on the mast cell stabilizers, I was taking prescription pain medicine. Now I only take an occasional Tylenol. A very big improvement!

I also believe that Cromolyn has helped a lot with my depression. It took several months for this to happen. If I skip a dose, I will feel emotional the next day. I will go into more detail in the chapter about Grief.

I am I completely healed? No. But am I able to leave the clean room? Yes! Is this the best I'm going to be? I hope not! I have lots of room for improvement. I am slowly adding vitamins to my diet. I know that my diet is lacking, so I need some supplements. Finding ones I don't react to has been a challenge. Hopefully, six months from now I will be even healthier!

When taking Cromolyn, remember to follow the directions. Dilute it in a cup of water. Take it on an empty stomach, two hours after eating. Wait 20 to 30 minutes before eating. It is challenging because you have to schedule all your meals and snacks around your Cromolyn doses, but it is well worth it.

Ordering Cromolyn through mail order can be downright frustrating. I think I had a small melt down on the phone with Express Scripts because my recent purchase was completely messed up. I paid for a 90-day supply, but only received an 18-day supply. I paid $500 for 18 days' worth of Cromolyn. As you can imagine, I was livid. I called and spoke to several people who all told me it was not their mistake because it was written for 720 ml instead of 720 vials. I was on the phone with the doctor's office when this was sent over. She definitely typed vials. This happened again when I called to have them send over another prescription. Something in someone's system is changing the vials to ml or no unit of measurement at all. I don't know if it is the doctor's computer or the computer system at Express Scripts. Either way, I'm the one paying for the problem. The pharmacist told me to have the doctor make sure the quantity was correct (which she did) and to write in the note section that the order is supposed to be a 90-day supply. This will help them if there is no unit of measurement in the script. If you pick up your medicine, I strongly suggest you count it before you leave. If you get it through mail order, call before they ship it and confirm that it is the correct amount. Feel free to learn from my expensive experience!

I have been on Cromolyn almost three years. Although it was hard to start, I do believe it is the best medicine I am on. I tell everyone I LOVE my Cromolyn, because I can't imagine where I would be without it!

There are several holistic approaches to many illnesses, for this one as well. For me, personally, a healthy diet was not enough. H1 and H2's alone were not enough. That is when the mast cell stabilizers were added. I can honestly say I would love to be able to take fewer medicines. I hope I will be well enough to drop a few someday. For now, I am thankful that the medicine is available.

I do know there are people who do well with a holistic approach and that is great. Would I ever suggest someone stop their medicine and try a holistic approach? No. Never. That could be dangerous. This is something that needs to be determined by the patient and their doctor.

The other day I read a question from one of the forums. A friend of mine has been taking care of her teen daughter who has several conditions including MCAS. She wanted to know if there were any supplements that could treat her daughter; she wanted to try to get her off all of the medicines. Knowing that she had just started Cromolyn, I immediately responded to please allow the medicine time to work. I recommended a low histamine diet, as well. I am not against supplements and healthy diets. In fact, I am all for them, but with this condition, you can't stop one thing and throw new things at it. You have to stop a medicine slowly and start one at a time... slowly. You have to give the medicine time to work.

Now this mom is a great mother. I have seen her live this struggle with her daughter. She posts her updates. This disease is horrible to have, but I can't imagine having to watch my child go through it. I have no doubt that the helplessness she and other parents must feel on a daily basis is overwhelming. It takes so long to get stabilized. It is hard to be patient.

There is conflicting advice on the internet. There are people who mean well who talk about their success stories of going off all medicine. This can be upsetting when improvement on the medications is so slow. We have to remember that every one of us is different. Our symptoms are different. Our bodies are different. Some of us have hives and diarrhea while some of us have severe reactions that require us to have an emergency medicine line-up. We are all at different places in our illness. Some of us cannot get to a stable place without the H1s, H2s and mast cell stabilizers. There are some lucky people who can. I just want the lucky people to remember some of us do require the medications to live and to function.

I once read that someone meditates during anaphylaxis instead of taking medication. I will NEVER do this. I believe this is very bad advice. If you are in anaphylaxis, take the appropriate medication, get medical attention and then pray or meditate. Meditating or praying can calm you down. This is a great thing, because stress can and will make it worse, but don't think this is just something you can overcome if you concentrate enough. True anaphylaxis is like a train barreling down the tracks without breaks. Very rarely will it stop on its own, you have to stop it.

I know with every medicine there are side effects, but without them I was having anaphylaxis several times a week. That is extremely hard on the body, so I have to choose the best way to get my disease under control and right now it is with medication. When I become extremely stable for some time, a more holistic approach might be a route to investigate.

Interestingly, I read that vitamin C can be a mast cell stabilizer and a degranulator based on the amount you take. You should take no more than 750 milligrams a day. Also, slow release vitamin C is recommended. I could not find slow release vitamin C, so I cut mine up and take it throughout the day.

Recommended treatment for mast cell disorders:

http://www.ncbi.nlm.nih.gov/pmc/articles/PMC3069946/table/T5/

Chapter 10: My Experience With Antihistamines

"Experience is one thing you can't get for nothing."

Oscar Wilde

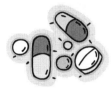 My experience with antihistamines has been interesting. Who knew that a little pill that is supposed to stop an allergic reaction could cause an allergic reaction? Well, through much trial and lots and lots of error, I have learned quite a few lessons and am happy to share the lessons I learned. Remember, however, that since we are all different with different reactions, what works for me won't necessarily work for you.

H1s are the antihistamines that block seasonal allergies like Allegra, Zyrtec, and Claritin.

H2s are the antihistamines marketed at reducing acid in the stomach. Pepcid and Zantac are actually antihistamines...who knew?!

I was on several combinations of H1s and H2s for months trying to find the right fit for my body. Finally, I have figured out through trial and error that Allegra and Zantac work best for me. I was on Zyrtec for several months and became allergic to it. I don't even know how this happens, but it does! This is where you have to take the time to figure out what combination will work for you, with your doctor's guidance. I consider these medications "maintenance medications". My "emergency" medication is Benadryl. I have actually reacted to Benadryl, but it wasn't the drug, it was the inactive ingredients in the Benadryl. First it was the red dye in the pink pills, then it was the ingredients in the liquid dye free. I have found that the Liquid Dye Free Caplets work best for me, they are much cleaner than the dye free liquid.

It is best to use your "emergency" medicine for emergencies only. This way, they remain effective. I have taken both Atarax and Benadryl as emergency medication. Atarax was my emergency medication for almost a year, but then it started causing the emergency! After that I switched to Benadryl.

Here are some lessons I learned:

Lesson 1-

Try to find "clean" antihistamines-the fewer the ingredients the better.

Lesson 2-

Try to find antihistamines with oxide dyes, not man-made dyes. For example, a man-made dye will have a number after the color. Red 40 and Yellow 10 are man-made dyes. Oxide blends come from the earth and are usually tolerated better.

Lesson 3–

Buying generic will sometimes help and sometimes hurt. This is where it gets tricky. I have found that with Zyrtec, Allegra and Zantac I have to have the name brand. With Claritin and Pepcid I actually did better with the generic brand.

I bought generic Allegra and had two days of itching so bad I thought I would lose my mind. Allegra is kind of expensive, but I have found the name brand to work well and after the experience with the generic, I will never go back. Generic Zantac has a lot of man-made dyes so I just stuck with the name brand. For the drugs that I found work okay with the generic, I stick with the same generic. I never go to different stores and by their store brand because every store will have a different formula and different ingredients. So, bottom line...this takes us to lesson 4.

Lesson 4-

If you buy generic and it works for you, stay with that particular brand. Don't buy the generic from different stores due to different ingredients. I buy my generic brands from Sam's Club, no other place.

Lesson 5-

If it works, keep it. Don't change it.

Lesson 6-

You can have an allergic reaction to an antihistamine- "mind blowing here".

Lesson 7-

You can have a life-threatening allergic reaction to an antihistamine- "bigger mind blowing".

Lesson 8-

Go slow. Don't change your antihistamine every three days. You have to try it for at least five to seven days to see if it is working. By all means, if you have a bad reaction, stop it immediately and call your doctor.

Lesson 9-

Start one at a time. Change one at a time. This goes for all medications. Never start two at the same time. You have to be able to tell what the medicine is doing for you. If you start more than one at a time you don't know which is doing what!

Lesson 10-

Carry them with you everywhere.

Chapter 11: Courage

"Courage is resistance to fear, mastery of fear, not absence of fear."

Mark Twain

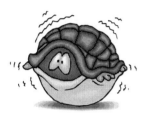 Triggers, triggers everywhere. Having severe reactions limits where I can go. Some might say that I need to find some courage and not worry about where I go. People who live with mast cell disorders would say getting out of bed every day is quite the display of courage! Don't let other people tell you what is safe. Be cautious and figure it out own your own.

Church and the movie theater or any enclosed building with a large number of people is especially hard. I am at a point where I am trying to go to these places. If I am having a bad day, by all means, I will not try. But, here lately I want to go more places. I just have to choose wisely.

We used to go to the movies a lot! We enjoyed the smell of the popcorn, and the excitement of the evening. When I first got sick I could not make it an hour at the theater before needing to run to the bathroom. Most of the movie was spent in the bathroom. As time moved on and as I got more stable I noticed that I actually made it through the first half of the movie. It was the second half that I was missing. Eventually, I could make it through the whole movie, but still the environment causes distress and sometimes diarrhea. I have even noticed my eyes swollen the next day.

Now there are a few things my husband and I have done to be able to go to the movie occasionally. One is to always wear a mask. This helps with perfume and cologne. Timing seems to be the most important. If you time it right, you can actually be one of a few people in the theater-that is usually our goal. That means you have to wait several weeks after the release of a movie. That's okay! We don't go often, but every once in a while it is a nice treat. (Pre-medication helps here!)

We have started attending a nearby church. It is a very large church. Large church means a lot of people. A lot of people means a lot of fragrance, perfumes, colognes, shampoo, conditioner, body wash, body spray, hairspray, soap, detergent and fabric softener. Think about all the products a single person uses in the morning. Take that number and multiply it by 300 people and what you have is an overwhelming amount of fragrance. I usually wear two to three medical masks and take Benadryl just to go to Sunday morning service. I think in the future we will look for a smaller church with fewer people.

My husband and I have stopped attending the dinner theater that we enjoyed. A lot of older people attend the dinner theater; older people tend to wear stronger perfumes. It was an unavoidable loss, a decision we had to make.

Stores can be full of triggers. Especially on the weekends when there are crowds of people. This is another activity that you just take for granted when you are healthy. To avoid the crowds we try to shop at the stores on off days, days that are less busy.

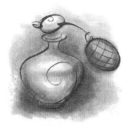 Environmental triggers like fragrance are a fast working trigger for me. Fragrance is a mast cell degranulator. As soon as I breathe it in, it starts a reaction. The mast cells open up and send out histamines and the histamines cause the symptoms to start. Flushing usually starts first which is often followed by diarrhea. Itching comes next-usually my eyes, feet or palms. After that, my throat starts to swell. This is where the fight or flight response would happen, but I have trained myself to remain as calm as possible.

Once the swelling has started, I know that I am having an anaphylactic reaction. My heart starts beating faster. This is the body's way of trying to compensate for what is going on inside. The blood vessels are starting to dilate and the blood pressure is dropping. This is all part of the anaphylaxis. This is frightening! I can minimize my fear by controlling where I go and being prepared when it happens. Notice I said "when" and not "if". I prepare by carrying my emergency medicines everywhere I go. At all times, I have with me two EpiPens, Benadryl, and Zantac (this is an H2 blocker). When a reaction starts, I remove myself from the trigger. I take one Benadryl. If the reaction continues, I take the second Benadryl, followed by the Zantac and EpiPen if needed. All this over perfume! So in the morning, when you are putting on your favorite perfume or cologne and you are considering going with two squirts-please, please go with one!

Other environmental triggers can include molds, dust mites, pet dander, heat, vibration, pressure, and new construction.

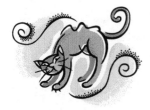

Mold, dust mites and pet dander are all known allergens, so I will skip to heat. Heat from the sun, heat from the bath water, heat from any source can cause degranulation. Heat is not a trigger for every person, but it is a known degranulator. Vibration from travelling in a car or in a plane and pressure from holding a child can cause degranulation.

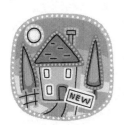

New construction is a quick degranulator for me. This is where a lot of formaldehyde is found along with many other V.O.C.s.

We joined a small group at church. I was excited to make some new friends. If ever I needed friends, it was now! We met with all of the group members and made plans for our next meeting. We planned a nice pitch-in type meeting. I made something I knew I could eat and would enjoy. Off we went. I was very upset when we arrived and could tell the house was new. But I had been on mast cell stabilizers for a while and I was bound and determined to have a good evening. Unfortunately, reality and what we plan can be quite different. By the time we left I had taken 2 Benadryl. We were there almost an hour and a half. I couldn't even go an hour and a half. My Benadryl was no match for the new construction. I reluctantly wrote a letter to the group leader explaining that even though we had a wonderful time I would not be able to attend any longer.

I have read that it take six years for the VOCs (Volatile Organic Compounds) to burn off in a newly constructed area or home. If you think of all the chemicals used in the building process it makes sense that it could be a problem.

I stay away from newly constructed homes, stores and restaurants. Luckily, I can tell pretty quickly when I walk into a building if it is going to be problematic for me.

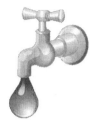

Another trigger that you don't think of right away is water. I was having trouble with all kinds of water- bottled water, the reverse osmosis water and tap water. I actually became very distressed about this. I wasn't drinking anything other than water. To react to the only thing you're drinking is pretty scary. I was told to try distilled water without minerals. It is the cleanest water available. Some will argue that you need the minerals in the water, which is true, but they could be causing issues. So start basic. You can always add the minerals in later. You can purchase distilled water at most stores. Baby water will contain fluoride, so steer clear of that.

I am not a fan of bottled water, except for the water in glass bottles. (Although the distilled water does come in gallon plastic jugs.) Just to be safe, I have removed all plastics from my house. I drink only from glass, because I believe that the plastics can leach into your food and drinks. This could be a trigger too!

Stress, exercise and sex can also be a mast cell degranulator.

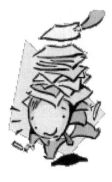

Stress is a huge trigger for many. I know for me, if something stressful happens, I can break out in hives and have diarrhea all in a matter of minutes. Now that I know what is going on. I can see the impact that stress has on my body. Trying to control the environment and cut down on stress can help tremendously. I recommend that.

If you have an extremely stressful job, consider looking for a less stressful job. Being healthy is by far more important than a job.

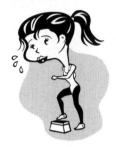

Exercise is a trigger. Honestly, I was so sick that I considered putting on my pajamas exercise! Now I am able to exercise at a slow pace. To me, at this point, any movement is good. I have a mini trampoline that I use to rebound on. I have read that rebounding (jumping up and down) will help clean out the lymphatic system. I need all the help I can get, so I try to jump a little throughout the day- a little in the morning, a little in the afternoon. By evening the only thing I'm going to jump on is the couch.

By eliminating triggers one by one, you can eventually get to a point where you can see how things affect you. Don't get discouraged. This process can take time-lots of time. If you are careful and diligent, clarity will come.

It took almost 8 months for me to be able to watch a two hour movie in the living room of my house. Honestly, I don't know if it was the mold, formaldehyde or if I was having problems with our pets. We re-homed some of our pets but ended up keeping three dogs and a cat.

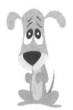

I found a fabulous home for one of my Pomeranians, but it was heart-breaking to see her go. Thank you, Mary, for giving Roselynn a home and loving her so much. I know she is in good hands and that helps a lot. Also, thank you for taking the time to stop by and visit me while I was sick. That was very nice and appreciated.

I had plans to re-home the other dogs, but I just couldn't do it. We thoroughly enjoy our pets. Our idea of a great time is watching one of the dogs play with a new toy. They are part of our family, so I couldn't do it. I struggled with this for months. On bad days I still struggle with this. My clean room is a pet free zone. My oldest dog Riley sat outside my clean room door for almost a year, just waiting for me to come out. How can I send her away when all she wants out of life is to see me?

If I had proof that re-homing the animals would help me, then I would. The proof will only come after they are gone and my health may not improve. I just can't bear the thought of their little faces when they are carted off from the only home they have even known. They are getting older so their years are limited. The plan as of today is to let them live out their days here in their happy home and not get any new pets. The thought of a day when I don't have a pet makes me sad. I don't look forward to the day when I will have to say goodbye to the last pet we own. Because of this disease, I have to consider the possibility that I will be physically healthier without a pet, but I'm just not ready to go down that road. They bring me joy, and when you are ill, an animal can make all the difference. They can brighten your day and put a smile on your face.

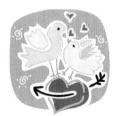 I have listed sex as a trigger. Now this is one trigger we should not have to eliminate. I figure that I have given up so much and there are some things I am unwilling to give up. With some research and determination, I have found a way to work around this issue. It is recommended by the top Mast Cell specialist to take an H2 blocker twenty minutes before engaging in sexual activates. For extra safety I will take an H1 blocker as well. These blockers help block the mast cells from degranulation during climax. How do you know if sex is a trigger for you? Flushing, hives, nausea and crying were my big clues. Luckily, not anaphylaxis! It was

kind of hard to convince my husband how much I enjoyed our time together when I was sobbing and trying not to puke. Poor guy-talk about mixed messages..."no, you are great, sob, sob, I have to throw up now!"

Remember, I am only an expert on me, so there may be some other symptoms that I have not listed. It is actually hard to find information on mast cells and sex! Determination pays off in this area.

Chapter 12: Lessons Learned

"Good judgment comes from experience, and experience comes from bad judgment."

Rita Mae Brown

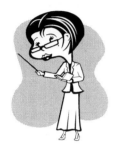 Experience is a brutal teacher.

A few summers back my daughters and I met my husband for lunch. We went to a restaurant close to his work. This restaurant is famous for their hamburgers. The restaurant boasts of all fresh meat, no additives or preservatives. As I mentioned before, there are only a few places that I can go and eat safely. I have eaten at this particular restaurant five or six times. So I feel like I'm fairly safe. I ordered a hamburger plain. When I got the hamburger it came out with lettuce (which I can eat), pickles (no), and tomatoes (huge no). My family suggested I take it back. I should have taken the sandwich back, but you know...you don't want to bother people; you don't want to accuse them of making it wrong; we'd already waited several minutes to get the food-the list is long. So I just picked all those topping off and started eating. I was half-way through when I realized that my sandwich also had "special" sauce on it. It was soaked into the bun. My family continued to tell me to take it back. But now half the sandwich is gone. I would look ridiculous taking back a half of sandwich and insisting on getting a whole new one! So I took the bun off. Now I am eating a topless sandwich. This is getting less appetizing by the minute!

I really, really wish I had listened to my family. On this day I had what I would call a delayed reaction. I was fine right after I ate the sandwich. I was fine kissing my husband goodbye. I was on the interstate for about ten minutes, when I felt the tightening in my throat. Now I'm not freaking out because this has happened so many times. So I started drinking water. Water is very helpful in flushing the body. A few minutes later I realized that the swelling was continuing and I asked my daughter to get in my bag and get a Benadryl. I took the Benadryl and the swelling continued. So I told my daughter to give me a Zantac, which is an H2 blocker. After taking the H2 I started getting nervous. I pulled off the interstate, took another Benadryl and told my daughter she had to drive. This was an "angry" reaction. I was wondering if I should go to the ER or just try to make it home. After a few minutes I felt like I couldn't hold my head up. That was either anaphylaxis or the Benadryl making me feel so bad. Usually it takes a little longer to go to sleep with the Benadryl. I made it home and took a three hour nap. I woke up with swollen eyes but my throat was not swollen any longer. It took two full days to recover from the incident. I had some kidney pain and all over pain the following days. This is one of the times that I can look back and think I probably should have used the epi pen and gone to the E.R. Actually, I've had several of those incidents. So for this reason I printed out an anaphylaxis chart and follow the directions on the paper. It is better to be cautious.

What I learned from this experience is that you cannot assume anything. My reaction was not from me just trying something but from assuming that it was a safe place to eat and that I was okay. Usually it IS a safe place to eat, but I will always, always check before I eat. I will no longer assume that the sandwich is what I ordered. In fact, it is probably best to assume that it is not what I ordered and be pleasantly surprised when it comes out correctly. Since then we have dubbed the sauce, "the sauce of death."

The sauce of death is actually a Thousand Island dressing. Let me walk you through how many ways this dressing is horrible for some people with mast cell disorders and salicylate sensitivity.

Its base commonly contains mayonnaise and can include olive oil, lemon juice, orange juice, paprika, Worcestershire sauce, mustard, vinegar, cream, chili sauce, tomato puree, ketchup or Tabasco sauce.

Lemon juice, orange juice, Worcestershire sauce, mustard, vinegar, chili sauce, tomato puree, ketchup and Tabasco sauce are ALL high in histamines or can be a mast cell degranulator. Paprika is the highest salicylate spice there is. I have gone into anaphylaxis by eating paprika alone.

It also typically contains finely chopped ingredients, which can include pickles, onions, bell peppers, green olives, hard-boiled egg, parsley, pimento, chives, garlic, or chopped nuts (such as walnuts or chestnuts).

Of the chopped ingredients, the pickles are high in histamines and the nuts can be a mast cell degranulator. The green olives are high in Salicylates. Garlic and onions do bother some people as well.

This is a horrendous list of degranulators, histamines and Salicylates. This dressing might need to be avoided by people with Mast Cell Disorders.

I was hesitant to go back to the restaurant after this incident. I did finally agree to go back, but I went back using good judgment that I had gained by the experience, I had learned from my bad judgment!

Chapter 13: Knowledge

"A little knowledge that acts is worth infinitely more than much knowledge that is idle."

Khalil Gibran

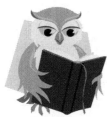 After two years of reactions in the house, finding and removing the mold from the duct work we finally ran all kinds of tests. We ran mold tests again along with radon, air quality and formaldehyde tests. I was convinced that there was mold still lingering. I felt something was causing my issues. I mostly felt it when I was downstairs. I suppose, again, I sounded a little crazy to some people. I felt fine in my clean room, but out of there I had a feeling of uneasiness, of something working against me. So I was ready to figure it out or move out!

It was the formaldehyde test that came back as the smoking gun. Our levels were three and a half times the recommended limit. You can find formaldehyde in all kinds of products in our homes, including treated wood, kitchen cabinets, or any kind of pressboard furniture.

Formaldehyde takes about 10 years to gas off. Our house is twenty years old, so after careful consideration and looking back at the time line, we realized that we had installed new laminate flooring about the same time I started reacting in the house. It was a very well-known brand. At the time we installed it we were unaware that it was full of formaldehyde. However, the company said it met the "high" safety standards.

Knowing the floor was the most likely culprit, we had to do what we had to do. We ripped up over a thousand dollars' worth of flooring. It was the only thing that made sense; the flooring was causing me these issues. I did a lot of research into formaldehyde and the problems exposure can cause. Bottom line-it is not good to be exposed to and can cause an array of allergies. I am pretty angry at this point because I feel, as a consumer, I should have been warned of the dangers. In fact, I called the company and asked where the warnings were. They would only say that the product meets safety standards.

My entire family went through about a week of detox- we were all sick. I looked this up and, to my surprise; this is something that can happen. It takes approximately 3 months for the levels to dissipate. After the 3 months we retested and the levels went back down to normal! So our educated guess about the laminate flooring was right. I have been able to spend more time in the entire house since we removed the laminate flooring. Looking back, I am seeing that a combination of things have contributed to my illness-a perfect storm, in essence.

My advice from this experience would be to get testing done as soon as possible. Don't wait two years as we did. I wasted two years being confined to the clean room when we could have removed the floor and I could have lived a more normal life. Two years I can't get back!! So yes, I would like to kick myself in the butt. What is done is done. Learn from my mistakes. Get those tests done sooner rather than later.

This advice also pertains to triggers. If you suspect a trigger, try removing it for a while. In fact, remove anything that could possibly be causing a problem, then walk through again and look for more suspects. It is far easier to remove everything and return one item at a time than to remove one item at a time.

Also, a good way to find out if your house is triggering you is to leave for a few days. It usually is very obvious upon returning after 4 or 5 days away if the house is a problem. I guess in a way it was easier for me to leave my house because I had no choice in the matter. I think it is harder to make the choice to leave. To me, a few days in a nice clean motel is better than an ER visit any day. Don't put off what you can do today to feel better tomorrow.

Here is the company that did our air quality test.

http://www.homeaircheck.com/

Chapter 14: Strange Triggers, Strange Reactions

"Science does not know its debt to imagination."

Ralph Waldo Emerson

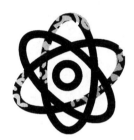

It seems to me as I become more and more aware of my triggers and avoid them, that when I do accidently come in contact with them the reaction is more severe. I have become so sensitive to fragrances that it is impossible to go into a store or public place without wearing a mask. A few months back we went shopping, the first time in a while that I had left the house. I was wearing an N95 mask, it must have leaked. I could feel a burning sensation in my lungs. This is and was my cue to leave immediately! I handed my cart off to my husband and got the car keys from him. I ran outside and ripped off the mask and took a few deep breaths. The store was small and there were lots of people shopping. The store also carried air fresheners, candles and incense. That was a bad combination. I got to the car and took one Benadryl because the pain went from burning to a stabbing sensation. It felt like I was being stabbed in the back with icicles. (Weird, I know.) The Benadryl eased the pain some. We skipped the rest of our plans to get me home - this happens a lot. By the time I got home I was not feeling right. I could smell that store on my clothes and my hair. I ran a tub of water and planned on taking an Epsom salt soak; this usually pulls some of the toxins out. I also needed to get that smell out of my hair. As I was taking my 20 minute soak, I started to feel woozy. It was then that I realized that sitting in deep water may not be the safest place to be. I was alone, everyone else was down stairs. So I immediately pulled the plug on the tub and let the water drain out before trying to get out of the tub. As soon as I got out I had to head to the toilet. I had a bowl movement, but not sure it would be considered diarrhea. Nausea started to set in. From there I got some clothes on and went to lie down. By now the pain is getting really, really bad. I am having a hard time taking deep breaths. I don't know if this is from the pain or if this is anaphylaxis. I have not been officially diagnosed with asthma, so I am at a loss for what to do. Now if I had been thinking straight, the right thing to do would have been to take another Benadryl and some Tylenol. Why didn't I think of that? Because when those mast cells trigger in your brain you don't think straight, even something as simple as a Benadryl and Tylenol.

The pain was really getting to the point that knew I had to do something. I considered using my Epi Pen, but my throat was not swollen or involved in any way. However, I was still having a hard time taking deep breaths. I did not know what to do. This was obviously an allergic reaction but the reaction was different than my "normal" reactions.

So we decided to go to the Immediate Care Center. Once again, Benadryl - take the stupid Benadryl!!! Take the Tylenol!! No - I still was not thinking straight. By the time we got to the Immediate Care Center, the pain was excruciating. It reminded me of being in labor, just higher up in my lungs. The doctor did not know what to do with me; she was truthful and said she had never seen an allergic reaction look like this. This is life with mast cell issues - you will hear that a lot. The next thing out of her mouth made me angry. She suggested that I was having a panic attack. I looked her square in the eye and said, "I am not upset or in a panic, I am in pain". I told her "I know what panic is and I was not having it". This is something so many of us hear - you have anxiety, you are having a panic attack. My stats are actually pretty good in this area; this was only the second doctor to suggest I was having anxiety. I cannot express the level of disappointment that each of these comments make us feel. We are reaching out for medical help and to be told that we are not having a medical emergency, but an emotional problem, is like slapping us in the face. We are trusting doctors to help us on a medical level. When I need counseling for an emotional problem, I don't go to a medical doctor, so why would I go to a medical doctor for an emotional issue? The truth of the matter is - the doctors are not familiar with mast cell issues. I am guessing we come across as a little crazy sounding. I mean I WAS explaining that I went into a store and it smelled bad and now I can't breathe...that does sound a little out there. Mast cell patients get this, they totally understand the fact that a smell can take you down, and down fast. This doctor didn't understand that fact. She has been taught to look for horses and not zebras, she has been taught to look at the most common situations. So yes, she was trained to recognize anxiety, and not a mast cell reaction. Where does that leave us? This leaves us in a very sticky situation because anxiety IS a symptom of anaphylaxis. So no matter what, there is always an element of anxiety.

When I have my normal reaction, I am prepared. I use my epi pen and I go to the ER with my nice detailed Emergency Folder. There is a chapter about the Emergency folder and its importance later in the book.

I try to stay as calm as possible for a couple of reasons. The number one reason I stay calm - it helps the mast cell reaction. The number two reason - if I am calm, then the doctors don't automatically assume I am having anxiety. This was not my normal reaction, so I think I may have been taken off guard and I was in a lot of pain.

She told me that they usually reserve the Epi for people who are in life-threatening situations, and I did not appear to be in one. Not knowing what to do with me, she gave me three options: One - she would give me epi; Two - I could go to the emergency room or; Three - she could give me that Benadryl and Tylenol that I forgot to take. I told her as I got in my purse and popped a Benadryl that I would go home and take my Tylenol; I knew the inactive ingredients in mine. I took the Tylenol as soon as I got home and the pain lasted for about 15 minutes. I was rolling around the bed, it hurt so much. Finally, the pain subsided and I had relief, but then I began to vomit for what seemed like 15 minutes. I grabbed my Epi Pen and was ready to go. I told my husband that I could not do this all night...it needed to stop. I gave it a few minutes and my body finally calmed down. I did take the advice from the doctor at the Immediate Care Center to call my specialist and make an appointment and get a plan in place. I was also told by this doctor not to come back to the Immediate Care Center, but to go to the hospital when I am in anaphylaxis. I am guessing she doesn't want to deal with this craziness and the hospital is more equipped to deal with anaphylaxis and anything else that goes along with it!

The next day, when I was feeling better, I posted my about my incident with the fragrance at the store and what followed and I questioned people about the use of the Epi Pen in a situation like this. After all, these people are the real experts - the ones who live with this day in and day out. Many said what I was thinking - that two or more systems were involved and they thought it was, in fact, anaphylaxis without throat swelling. They stated I should have used my Epi Pen. I know a woman who only has this kind of anaphylaxis, she never has swelling. It is unusual but it happens. I had some who stated that they don't use the Epi Pens unless they have trouble breathing or swelling of the throat.

So there you have it folks, even the experts, the ones who live with this, have a different opinion about how to deal with this disorder. No wonder the doctors don't understand and know what to do with us. I did see my specialist and she stated that she didn't think it was an Epi Pen worthy situation. However, looking back I am certain that the epinephrine would have helped avoid the two or three hour ordeal. Was it life-threatening? Maybe not since I didn't pass out, but how do you Epi after you pass out? It is very hard to live with something and know the dangers of it and yet not know how or when to treat yourself.

"When you hear the sound of hooves, think horses, not zebras."

This is a phrase taught to medical students during their training. In medicine, the term "zebra" is used in reference to a rare condition or disease. Doctors are taught to assume that the simplest explanation is most likely correct. Therefore doctors learn to expect common conditions.

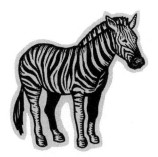

"I look for zebras because other doctors have ruled out all the horses." — Dr. Gregory House

I wonder how many of us have wished we could see Dr. Gregory House. I dreamed of seeing him, even though he was a fictional character. I was convinced he could help me! He did help a mastocytosis patient in season 8 episode 1!

Another strange reaction occurred when I was riding in my husband's car. We were in the car about 10 minutes when my throat started getting that feeling. I told him I was having issues and I got the Benadryl out and took it. I asked him what was in the car. His response surprised me. He told me that a day or two before he had carried a piece of treated lumber. Remember, treated lumber usually has formaldehyde. I was reacting to what used to be in the car! This was a good lesson in what to carry in the car that I drive and ride in the most. I don't carry anything that could make me trigger.

One of my biggest triggers was a mystery for a while. I believe it was from getting a new refrigerator. That day I was removing all the food from the old refrigerator and stacking it in the kitchen. My husband was outside working on repairing the fence. The fence had some mold on it and I had reacted to it earlier in the summer. I did my best to stay away from the scraping and repair work. It was very important that Dan put his clothes it the washer immediately after he came in from the working on the fence. The delivery of the refrigerator came several hours early, without notice. When this happened Dan just came in and we didn't think about the mold that he had been scraping off the fence. It didn't cross our minds to have him change clothes. We did think about the new appliance and the off gassing so we bought a floor model hoping that the newness had already gassed off. When they took out the old refrigerator, nasty stuff was leaking out and we were mopping it up with whatever cleaner we could find the fastest. I washed out the inside of the new one with a little bit of bleach water. I usually do okay with bleach water. We had a bunch of frozen foods that were not going to fit into the new freezer, so we had variety meal with all sorts of goodies. Some of them, I'm guessing were not safe for me to eat. I also remember eating a tomato that day and a tiny bit of very lightly sauced pizza. (Today I can't eat tomatoes or tomato products at all and have even reacted to the juice left after removing them from my salad.) Even after all of these things I seemed fine. I went and took my Epsom salt soak.

After that we were watching TV in the clean room, when all of a sudden I could not swallow. Freaky! I popped out of bed and started drinking water and took a Benadryl. No relief, so I took the second Benadryl. Still no relief, this was an intense reaction. I knew I needed to Epi and head to the Emergency Room, so that is what I did. Amazing how fast the Epi Pen works! By the time we got to the hospital I felt much, much better. They asked me what I thought caused the reaction. I could not give them a straight answer. I had been exposed to numerous triggers with nothing happening and then when I was safe in my clean room, I reacted. It did not make any sense, even to me. I do remember smelling smoke from a fire pit right after it happened and when we went to the car. So that is what I told them at the hospital. I think smoke from the fire pit caused it. Because, really, if I told them that the new appliance or moldy clothes did it...well that would just sound crazy!

Keeping the clean room clean requires us to block off the central air and heat in that room. So in the winter we use a beautiful electric fireplace. I truly enjoy using the fireplace. In the summer we use a window air conditioner. As of today we are on number 3. The first one did okay, but turned out to be too small for the room. This resulted in a hot room most of the time. Remember - heat can be a trigger. So we took that little air conditioner out in the fall determined to buy a much bigger one for next summer. When summer came around that is exactly what we did! We found a much bigger one and my husband lugged that thing up the stairs. We wrestled it out of the box and finally got it up in the window. Being that is was an upstairs window made me nervous; there was no way to hold it up from the outside while installing it! I had visions of the big thing just falling and crashing to the ground. So with lots of slow adjustments we got the thing in right. We used a piece of UNTREATED wood in the top of the window to prevent the window sash from moving up. Bravo, we have cool air and lots of it! We are happy as clams!

It was a long, hot summer; in fact we had a drought. There were 'no burn' orders and 'no watering the lawn' orders from the city. Hot, hot, hot! So we were happy with our decision to buy the larger air conditioner. When fall rolled around, we looked at that big thing and each other and decided to leave it in. Maybe wrap the outside in plastic. It was so huge, and so nerve-racking to get it in, not to mention that we didn't know where to store it? The first answer would be in the garage. But would it stay "clean" enough for us to use again in the clean room? So we went with leaving it in the window. We did put some plastic sheeting up to the window to block out the cold of winter. This way we even saved a step, in the spring. This has always been a personal motto of mine...do it this way, and "save a step"! Don't put it in the sink, put it in the dish-washer and save a step...you get the idea.

Spring rolled around and, voila, take down to plastic and we are ready to go! How easy was that? When it started getting hot we just cranked that air conditioner up and we were ready to go! So as life is never dull for a person with a mast cell disorder...it wasn't long before I started trig-gering. When this happens I retreat to the clean room. So that's what I did, but for some reason, I didn't start to get better. In fact, I seemed a bit worse with each day I spent in there. So I got angry, which is a normal chemical re-sponse to my many mast cells, but I was also angry because I thought something had breached my clean room! Something has gotten in through the cracks in the door! I dragged myself out of bed and dusted the best I could and flopped back down in the bed. I didn't want to leave because think how much worse off I would be out of the clean room. It didn't make sense - I had dusted and cleaned all I could, so why was this happening? I had even dusted the surface of the big air conditioner and it wasn't even that dusty. I remembered that there is a little filter on the air conditioner that needs to be clean periodically. So I took the front off and looked at it thinking it must be full of dust! No- it was clean. So I have spent the last two years being a detective of everything. Seems like I am always trying to figure and backtrack to what could have caused this problem. I'm getting pretty good at it too, except this time I was stumped. I have cleaned everything. I have taken items out of the room that have been considered safe. We have done our best to eliminate anything that doesn't need to be in there. I don't get it. Retiring back to the bed, because all my energy has been spent cleaning every nook and cranny, I am an emotional wreck. My space of solitude has been soiled and I don't have a safe place any longer. Then it dawned on me that I haven't cleaned the inside of the air conditioner...I don't think you can even clean the inside of an air conditioner. But I was going to try! So I am trying to figure out how to take off the little air deflectors without breaking them. I am finding that they don't come off. So I grab a flash light. I decide to see if it even requires cleaning.

OH YEA, "Houston, we have a problem". Is it as bad as Apollo 13? For me, yes! Mold was growing in the air conditioner. Mold = anaphylaxis. I didn't know if I should shout for joy or cry! What a confusing situation. I ran and made a bucket of water with a little bleach. That little wind deflector that wouldn't come off, yes I ripped that thing right off. I was going to annihilate that mold and nothing was going to stop me, not even common sense! Now, we are all thinking at this point in the story of the air conditioner, that standing around with bleach water and trying to clean mold out of anything, is probably NOT the best idea. I do realize this now. For some reason, during a flare or trigger, it seems like the common sense or the ability to think straight is not an option. I even find it hard to figure out when to take meds at the right time. For this reason, I have made a chart on the wall - you can't argue with paper. The paper says if you can't swallow use the Epi Pen, don't sit there and try to reason with the paper that the Benadryl may kick in. Just follow the chart - it never wavers and it is always right. If I had a chart about cleaning mold with bleach it would say...Never clean mold, with anything.

During this whole process, I called my husband. I was shouting for joy and most likely crying at the same time. Again, my husband wins all awards for putting up with crazy stuff. His reaction, as usual, is calm and precise. "I will stop on the way home and buy a new one." Wow, I had not even thought of that. I was too busy ripping off the air deflector and throwing it across the room and cleaning with that bleach. Man, I love my husband. He totally gets it. He knows there is no point in trying to clean this crazy thing. He has been dealing with this crazy illness long enough to know it wins. It gets what it wants; it wants a mold free air conditioner.

It seems to me that we have been through many tribulations in our house. I was ready to move the first year with the flood and mold in the duct work. Then there were the high formaldehyde levels and, for the record, my husband says we can't count that because we brought that into the house. It was not the house. So I will give him that.

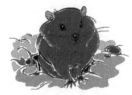 Our next tribulation came in the form of a little rodent. A vole – no, not a mole, a vole. It is an adorable little creature that looks like a hamster. It is shorter and fatter than a mouse. It is quick as lightening when it runs and they are very hard workers, I might add.

When the spring weather turned warm, I noticed an odor when I walked into the living room. I would walk around sniffing and asking, "Does anyone smell that?" Of course not, I have a nose that can smell something a mile away. This is something that is common with mast cell people, not all, but many are bothered by smell. Our sense of smell increases and we can smell things that others can't. As the days got warmer the smell got stronger. The day finally arrived when others could smell it. On the warmest day of spring, my daughter Emily told me she could smell it and described it as smelling like a urinal.

One afternoon I was in the stinky room and heard a scratching going on in the wall. Now I had a clue. I also remember Bethany coming home and saying it freaked her out when the cats just sat and stared at the wall, like they could see something she couldn't! So upon discussing these things with Dan, he mentioned he had heard the scratching late at night. We went outside to investigate and found lots of dirt on the front porch. We looked at each other and neither of us had moved the dirt there. So now we knew we had a problem. We thought they were mice. We stood there awhile just waiting and watching. Nothing happened. Over the next few days I did see little gray streaks of fur running back and forth outside. They were fast and very seldom did you get a good look at them. I hated to trap them, but the warmer it got, the smellier the house got. It started to bother me and seemed to trigger me. I found it harder and harder to sit in the living room.

Unfortunately, they built a metropolis in our wall. They had ample space to make their homestead. We are not certain how long they were in the wall, perhaps six months.

Before long, I was sitting everywhere but the living room. We called out an exterminator and explained our situation. He looked around and asked me what they looked like. I told him they were grey and actually kind of cute. He pointed out the tunnels in the landscaping. He said, "mice don't build tunnels like those". They had a whole metropolis outside too! He said they are called voles. They are shorter and fatter than mice - I think that is why they look so cute, they remind me of hamsters. He told me that they have been gathering bird seed from the bird feeder for months. Setting out traps would be pointless because they most likely have enough food to last a long time. He said they really don't deal with voles. So we were left to deal with them ourselves. So we found their point of entrance and set a bucket under it. If the vole came out of the house they would fall into the bucket. We then took them over near the pond to let them rebuild there. In total we caught around 36 of them.

We figured we had caught enough to call in the contractor to make the repairs to the wall. They would need to take the drywall down, remove the soiled insulation, Kilz the wood to prevent any other stink and rehang new drywall. I had spent several days in the clean room because of the smell. I knew that tearing the wall open would result in me needing to stay there for a few days to be safe. We called a contractor; he was to come out on Friday. So the Thursday before, we moved all the furniture out of the living room and into the dining room. We then hung plastic all over, blocking off door ways to prevent drywall dust from going everywhere. The plastic sheeting itself had a bad odor, it smelled like something burning. I decided to let Dan handle it and went to the clean room. I was afraid of the plastic at this point. Dan had taken off work on that Friday to be available to the contractor, because I was staying put where I was safe. Friday when I woke up it was obvious I had reacted to the plastic, my face and eyes were swollen. So I just dealt with it. Several hours passed and the contractor was late. Dan called several times and there was no answer. He left several messages, but received no response. Unfortunately, he never showed up. I was trying not to become hysterical but nothing is easy with a mast cell disorder. I am reacting to the plastic that is all over, but should we take it down? We need it up. I am sure I was a grump, but I was really ticked off. Why do people say they are going to show up and then don't. Let your "Yes" be "Yes" and your "No" be "No". We started making phone calls and most people were two weeks out. Oh my goodness, that means I will have to be in that room for at least two weeks. I would be stir crazy! Thankfully, we did get a call back from a local guy who was able to make it out in 5 days. I could do 5 days! So we left the plastic sheeting up for the 5 days. We figured I had a hard time downstairs with the vole smell anyway, plus putting up new sheeting would stink even more. So I stayed in the clean room. The handy man showed up on time, and Dan sent me pictures of the findings! The voles had quite a home!

Sometimes when bad things happen they happen for a reason, turns out that our window was leaking and we didn't know about it. The wood under the window was wet, not moldy yet, but indeed wet. So were the voles a blessing in disguise?

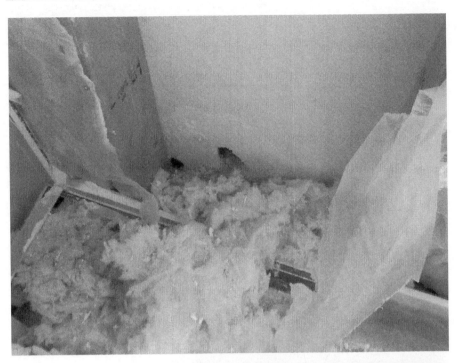

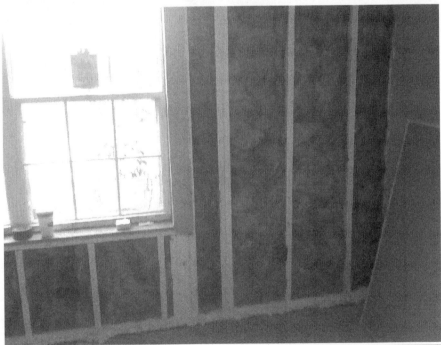

Other strange triggers:

Fake Leather furniture

New furniture

Fragrance of any kind

Cleaners of any kind

Smoke from a fire pit

Glues

Detergents

Fabric softeners

Dust

Molds

Vacuum cleaners

Make-up - foundation, eye liner, lip stick, eye shadow, etc.

Wet leaves in the fall

Books- book mold/dust

Garbage disposal (mold)

Memory Foam anything - mattress, pillow etc.

Sharpie markers

Ink on newspapers

Ink in magazines

Plastic cups

Plastic dishes

Mums - they are a member of the ragweed family

Toothpaste

Clothing dyes

Soap

Water (additives in water) -Distilled with no minerals works best for me.

Press board furniture - formaldehyde

Laminate flooring - formaldehyde

Vinyl flooring

Using hot water in the shower or bath

Sun

Heat

Cold

Friction

Vibration

Sex

Steam from cooking

Heat from cooking

Hormones

Stress

Anxiety

The process of eating and digesting food

Medications

Salicylates in products

Massage chairs/beds

Formaldehyde in clothes

Even an empty stomach

New Appliances

Plastic dishes

Ice cold drinks

Pain

Loud noises

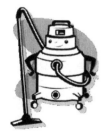 I would like to mention that I was having a hard time using the vacuum cleaner. Even though we don't have any carpet in the house, I found that using the vacuum we had just made me trigger. Doing lots of research I found one that I thought would be really safe. The Miele vacuum has several filters in it and it does an awesome job of eliminating dust particle from getting into the air. The lady at the store demonstrated it by using a particle measuring tool. I was impressed and sold on it. Now I can do some of the sweeping!

Miele website: The AirClean Filter System

"The outstanding filtration of Miele vacuum cleaners is the result of a filtration system consisting of the innovative Miele AirClean dustbag, a motor protection filter and a Miele exhaust filter. The way these components complement each other ensures that more than 99.9% of fine dust is filtered out. You can breathe again!"

http://www.mieleusa.com/Product/Vacuums

While we are on the topic of reactions, there are many drugs, chemicals and foods that are mast cell degranulators. Meaning when you consume these products they have a chemical reaction that makes mast cells open up. You don't have to have an allergy, they are just known degranulators. I have included this website for a detailed list. http://www.mastocytosis.ca/symptoms.htm

Chapter 15: Diets

"A crust eaten in peace is better than a banquet partaken in anxiety."

Aesop

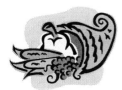 Anyone with a food allergy knows that a morsel of the offending food can be deadly. So you must train, and restrain yourself! A lot of people find their food allergies early in life and, from my perspective, this would be much easier than waking up one day and finding out you are "allergic" to most of your favorite foods. When you find the allergies early in life you don't know what you are missing, so to speak.

To complicate matters, with mast cell disorders you have allergic reactions to triggers and yet may or may not show IGE allergies to those triggers. In other words, all the blood work I had to test allergies shows that I am not allergic to anything and yet my body reacts like it is. The doctor said that I am "allergic to the world." However, I don't have test results telling me what to avoid. It is all trial and a lot of error figuring out what is what and how my body will react. I am mostly stabilized now, meaning my mast cell stabilizers are working and I know what to avoid and have been doing so, decreasing my incidence of anaphylaxis.

At one point I was told that I was intolerant to casein and to stay away from dairy. I was born with a stick of butter in one hand and an ice cream cone in the other! My mom has told me many times if a stick of butter was missing she would find what was left of it in my room under my bed with little teeth marks in it. So the idea of no dairy took a lot of work. That makes eating cereal hard and just think-how do you eat an OREO cookie without milk? Pizza is not pizza without melted cheese on it. Anyone who knows me can tell you that at any given moment I have 37 different kinds of ice cream in my freezer! I had a long struggle ahead of me.

I started exploring alternative milks such as almond milk and rice milk. Thinking about people squeezing the milk out of those little pieces of rice, wow that would be something else! I envisioned them milking them like little cows.

I started buying fake cheese from health food stores. I think it was made out of soy. I would make my little pizza with the fake cheese while the family was eating their gooey, bubbly mozzarella covered dish of deliciousness! I knew if I stuck to it, I would start to feel better. So I hung in there.

Unfortunately, I didn't really feel better. So I decided to alleviate all the chemicals from the products that I used daily. Working at the library I had access to many books on the subject. So I started buying all my products from the health food stores. My shampoo was made of lavender, my soap was mint and toothpaste was made of real cinnamon. Everything was all natural, no additives or preservatives. Everything was from a plant, from the earth, surely this would make difference. Oh, it made a difference all right. I went from being sick to being really sick, I just didn't know why at the time.

Being confined to my clean room, my environment was very controlled. I started to see a pattern, that I would break out in hives and my throat would swell after I brushed my teeth and used mouthwash. This was a huge clue! I remember a paper that the doctor had given to me listed mint. For months I had done research on different diets and allergies. The doctor had given me many different reading materials. I had to dig through piles of paper work to find it. Finally, digging it out from the pile I saw the word mint! It was a paper on Salicylate Sensitivity. I had no idea what a salicylate was or what it did. I think back how many times I had that paper, the answer, in my hands. Wow, that was eye opening. I started scouring the internet for anything to do with salicylates. I joined a few groups. I was so eager to figure out the answers.

Salicylates are in many of the products we use on a daily bases. Most soap, lotions, shampoos, detergents, fabric softeners, artificial colors, artificial flavors, preservatives and products with fragrances can contain salicylates. Aspirin is a salicylate because it is acetylsalicylic acid. This was starting to make sense. I remember having to go into the bathroom at work to change my shirt, because I could not stand the fabric softener that I have used for years.

The doctor gave me a low salicylate diet to follow. Unfortunately, salicylates are in most fruits, veggies and spices. This is why I had gone into anaphylaxis after the meal at the wedding and the dinner theater. Avoiding salicylates makes eating very difficult and eating healthy even harder!

All the natural products I was using were high in salicylates. At the time I had never heard of a salicylate. So instead of getting better I got worse in the beginning before making the connection to salicylates.

I stumbled upon a sad truth...sometimes healthy can be harmful. The almond milk was high in salicylates, so I was unintentionally making things worse by replacing my dairy products.

There are some theories that say you develop food allergies because of a "leaky gut". The theory states that food leaks out of the stomach and is considered foreign by the body. The body goes into attack mode and, boom, you have an allergy. I sometimes wonder if this is when I could have developed my salicylate sensitivity. I was changing my diet and all of my personal products, most of which all contained high salicylates. I was trying to eat very healthy, lots of fruits and veggies. I knew I was sick, so all natural was the obvious way to go. I have read from my salicylate sensitive friends that they think they became salicylate sensitive when they started juicing and went on a juice cleanse. Again, this would make sense based on the leaky gut theory. So take a note of that! Everything in moderation.

It would also stand to reason that if a leaky gut is the cause for many of these issues, then repairing or fixing a leaky gut would help. So I have done a lot of research about this. There are numerous products available on the market to help with the repair of the leaky gut. It is said you have to repair the mucus lining before taking probiotics. I believe Cromolyn has really helped repair my gut. It does sooth it. I am going to try the probiotics soon. The task will be to find a probiotic that is not high in histamines.

I am currently on a low histamine and a low salicylate diet. I have found that salicylates are my worst triggers. Salicylates are listed as a mast cell degranulator. I can't "cheat" with salicylates. Very high and high salicylates quickly cause my throat to swell. Salicylate sensitivity can make eating healthy incredibly hard. Thankfully, there are different levels of salicylates in different foods, which allow those of us with salicylate sensitivity some options, unlike a wheat allergy where wheat must be totally avoided. Salicylate levels fall into one of five categories: Very High, High, Moderate, Low, and Negligible. The majority of spices fall under very high or high. Most fruits are also considered high to very high. Exceptions are peeled pears, golden delicious apples, limes, bananas, mangos and pomegranates. Thankfully, there are more veggies to choose from, but most are not on my favorite list. Bamboo shoots and chokos are both veggies that are safe, but foreign to me. I don't have the slightest idea how to cook and eat a bamboo shoot, nor do I ever want to learn. I have no clue what a choko looks like or even how to pronounce it! Veggies that are lower in salicylates are white cabbage, cauliflower, brussel sprouts, celery, iceberg lettuce, potatoes, fresh asparagus and green beans.

My diet stays between low and moderate salicylates. Another thing to keep in mind with salicylates is that they stack. If I have several moderates, they can stack up to a high and I can react.

There are a few foods like limes and peanuts that are safe as far as salicylates go, but I can't eat them because they are mast cell degranulators and I react to them. Bananas are tricky as well because they are low in salicylates but can be high in histamines depending on the ripeness. It is best for me to avoid very ripe bananas. So I have to consider both the salicylate and the histamine content. That narrows the food options even more!

The crazy thing is that I can safely eat chocolate cake (depending on the chocolate) or cookies but can't eat most vegetables without needing Benadryl and sometimes Epinephrine. My chance of getting thin...is, well, pretty thin! I have learned the hard way that not all diets make you skinny!

I have been overweight since having children. I can say without a doubt, I am a bad dieter! I love to bake anything-cookies, cakes and bread. So REALLY, having to diet was, and still, is a challenge. For the first few months, I carried lists around with me. I soon came to realize to avoid preservatives, artificial colors and flavors; I would have to cook everything from scratch. I learned to read every ingredient list. Now, you would think it would be common sense, but I learned from experience to read the ingredient list before you eat the food. So many times I would think the food was fine only to have a reaction and then read the label. Apparently, I am hard-headed by nature.

When the family wanted something I couldn't have, I would make myself a steak dinner. I can eat steak, baked potatoes and green beans. So I eat this meal a lot! I have also gained weight—a lot! I am starting to come to terms with the diet, and I have learned to substitute ingredients. I am starting to lose some of the extra weight. I am trying to make better decisions with the choices I have.

Dieting like this makes it very hard to eat out. My husband has always loved to eat out. There are a few places I can go that don't use as many preservatives and cook from scratch. I guess in the long run we are saving money by not eating out and everyone else is kind of forced to eat healthier. A good rule to remember: "If you cannot pronounce it, don't eat it!"

Not all people with Mast Cell issues have salicylate sensitivity, but there is a small percentage who do. Many people have made improvements by removing gluten and/or dairy from their diets. The elimination diet is a good one to try. You basically eliminate everything but a few safe foods, then slowly add one in at a time. I believe this is the easiest way to see food triggers, but this was, by far, the hardest diet for me.

There is also the Rotation Diet. This is where you don't eat the same food consecutively; you eat the same food about every three days.

Most people who have a mast cell disorder do find that doing a low histamine diet benefits them. I have found it incredibly helpful for keeping me out of the bathroom.

Foods that are high in histamines cause gastro-intestinal distress...to say the least.

When mast cells degranulate, massive amounts of histamines escape and cause problems. Most of us are on antihistamines to limit the number of histamines that float around the body. The act of digesting food creates histamines. One of our fights is with histamines. Therefore, it is essential to be on a low histamine diet. Does it make sense to take antihistamines day and night and then go and eat histamines in every meal? NO! The funny thing is that I'm not sure most doctors are convinced about the value of a low histamine diet. I sure am. I can eat a food high in histamine and within a few minutes need to run to the bathroom and that is running, not walking fast or skipping.

 Meat is a big histamine source. Histamine starts growing as soon as an animal is slaughtered. So getting fresh meat is important. Histamines rise as meat cooks and continues to rise after cooking. Leftovers are not safe in the refrigerator and should be frozen. The freezing stops the histamine release. If you put your meat in the refrigerator, the histamines will continue to grow.

I have a crazy story about a high histamine food. This was early on when I didn't understand the way histamines grow. My daughter wanted to go and spend a few days with her friend at college. This was the first car trip since my diagnosis. I was weak and but wanted to do something normal. My husband was driving, so *all* I had to do was ride and stay alive. My daughter had helped me so much I wanted her to have some fun and get to see what living in the dorm was like. So we packed up and took the 5 hour trip. Now normal people think "what is the big deal?", but for "masto" people, leaving the house is a big deal. I knew physically I could not do a round trip in one day. That was not possible. So I booked a motel. Take a note here: while booking the motel I found one in a city that had a hospital because I was not completely stable. I didn't feel safe staying away from home. So knowing there was a hospital nearby gave me a little peace of mind. There was a cheaper one about 30 minutes away, but this is not the time to be cheap! I also called ahead and requested that they didn't use any air fresheners in the room. Staying in a motel can be hit or miss, depending on the cleaners used in the room and the detergents used in the bedding. Again, this is something you really have no control over so you get what you get so I always pack my own linens, just in case. Take another note: Always ask to inspect the room prior to accepting and paying for it. This way, if it is unacceptable, you can find another room or another motel. Yes, I learned this from experience too!

On the way home we found one of the few restaurants I can eat at. We had brunch, it was around 11. I couldn't eat all of my salad-it was too large. The salad had veggies and chicken on it. I asked to take it home. We boxed it up and that was that. We made a few stops on the trip home. We were not in a giant hurry to get home. Again, this is the first car trip we had made. So it was nice to feel normal and to try to forget for a few minutes that mast cells rule my life. About three hours later we left the cities and came to a more rural area of the trip. I was getting hungry. I knew there would not be a safe restaurant for miles. So I dug in the back seat and found my left over salad. Take a Note: Never dig in the back seat for a left over anything! Ahh, that salad hit the spot! It was as good then as it was earlier in the day.

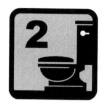 My Mmm Mmm's turned to Uhhh Ohh's really fast! Did I mention we were in the middle of nowhere? It was like a scene from National Lampoon's Vacation. I was about to explode. All we saw were corn fields and a train. In fact, we were stopped by the longest, slowest train on the planet. After what seemed like an hour, we hustled up the road and oh, thank goodness, we could see a gas station in the distance, halleluiah! As we got closer, it became obvious that the gas station was boarded up. I think I may have been tearing up at this point. We saw a business and I was desperate enough to go and beg someone to let me use their potty, but it was Sunday and it was closed too.

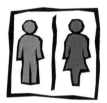 So, with much anticipation, we finally found a bathroom at a gas station. It was your normal, gross gas station, but at this point I didn't care. Dan parked and I did the shimmy run through the parking lot and through the gas station, still not sure why he didn't just drop me off. He parked the car on the side of the gas station. Why? Why are you parking the car 500 feet away from the door? I finally got to the bathroom and it was occupied, someone was in there. I am sure at this point I was jogging in place...please, please be done NOW! Finally, the occupant emerged. I may or may not have shoved the person out of the doorway when they walked out. I really have suppressed that memory. While I was washing my hands before leaving the bathroom, I looked up and was shocked that my face, neck and chest were completely flushed. I was red all over like Rudolf the Red Nosed Reindeer. I was kind of glowing. This was a little scary, but my throat was fine. When I got to the car I took some Benadryl and we headed home. I learned a very, very important lesson that day...never ever eat left overs that have been sitting in your car for even just a few hours. The salad was still cool in a Styrofoam container, but the

histamines were multiplying! I just didn't think about that. - Now I do.

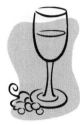 Alcohols and Teas are high in histamine naturally. They are also high in salicylates so it is best to for me to avoid these entirely. Coffee is a hit and miss for people and a no go for me. If you are able to consume coffee, freshly brewed is best. Avoid the instant and flavored coffees.

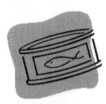 Fish start to grow histamines immediately after being caught. Unless you gut and cook your fish immediately after catching it, it is not recommended. All shellfish and canned fish are high in histamines.

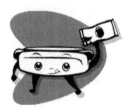 All processed meats including bologna, hotdogs, pepperoni and salami are high in histamines, as well as all pickled foods.

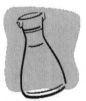 Fermented soy products, like soy sauce are not recommended. They are really high in histamines. I learned this after eating at a Japanese restaurant. I was telling my doctor about the event that took place and he looked at me and said "you can't eat things like that!" Well, now I know that. I didn't before but, yes, I can see that is problematic. I think he forgot to tell me about this or I totally missed the boat. Either way, I know now not to eat this.

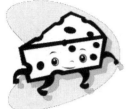

Other fermented food products- yogurt, yeast breads and cheeses are all high in histamines. I personally can't touch yogurt. I do great with homemade bread but I don't do great with cheese. I do okay with some cheeses that are not aged too long like mozzarella. I can't eat cheddar, as it is aged. I found this out one evening when I made some potato soup and put some cheddar cheese in it. We were eating dinner as a family and we all sat down to enjoy the soup. Mine didn't stay down very long and I ended up vomiting in the kitchen trash can. Unfortunately, for me, vomiting sometimes results in uncontrolled urination. (I blame this on the children.) This time was not an exception; I was vomiting and urinating while standing in the kitchen. Apparently my family is quite used to this kind of scenario as they just carried on eating their meal! It was dinner and a show!

One important fact worth repeating- Always freeze left overs! Left overs in the refrigerator WILL grow histamines. The freezing temperatures are the only thing that stops the histamine growth.

Another thing to consider is the way we prepare our foods. So yes, not only do you need to think about what you are preparing, but now you need to stop and think about how you are preparing your food, because the way you cook it does contribute to the histamine levels and to the growth of amines.

If you are cooking a pot roast in the crock pot, yum, that roast cooks slowly all day, roasting those potatoes, onions and carrots oh so slow. It also grows histamines the whole time! I learned this the hard way! I would make this fabulous pot roast and sit down to enjoy it, only to almost fall asleep in my plate! It took me several times of doing this to finally see the pattern. I was confused because they were all safe foods for me, so why did I feel so weird after eating my safe foods? It wasn't what I was eating; it was the way it was cooked!

Browning foods creates amines. Amines are a naturally occurring chemical; they are a result of the breakdown of protein or the fermentation process. They are a type of histamine. Every time I would caramelize onions and eat them I would want to take a nap during my meal. This is not normal! Again, after testing this a few times, I started to see a pattern. Once I saw the pattern I was determined to find an answer. Here is a link to learn more about amines.

http://aminerecipes.com/what-are-amines/

Since we are all so different and we all have differing triggers, it may be wise to start the elimination diet to "see" what triggers you have.

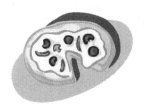 I asked my daughter the other evening what she wanted for dinner. She said "Pizza, but I know you can't have that." I responded "I can have pizza, without the sauce, and the sausage." She laughed and said "Mom that is called bread, not pizza". Hey, I call it pizza! With a little swapping out I can have my version of pizza!

I have found a great substitute for tomato sauce. It is called the Nomato sauce. You can use it in place of any kind of tomato sauce. It is low in histamines and moderate in salicylates! I have provided the recipe here for your enjoyment!

Basic Nomato Sauce (Tomato Free Tomato Sauce)

Ingredients:

Servings: 2

6 carrots, peeled and diced

1 small beet, peeled and diced

1 large onion, diced

3 celery ribs, diced **I leave the celery out because I am reactive to it.**

1 bay leaf, whole ***I don't use the bay leaf to keep the salicylate levels down.***

1 1/2 cups water

Directions:

1-Put everything in a covered pot, bring to a boil, reduce heat to simmer until veggies are soft.

2-Take out the bay leaf, blend well till smooth and use as you would tomato sauce, spicing appropriately for the dish you're using it in.

I make a double batch and freeze it-save a step!

http://www.food.com/recipe/basic-nomato-sauce-to-mato-free-tomato-sauce-359835?scaleto=2&mode=null&st=true

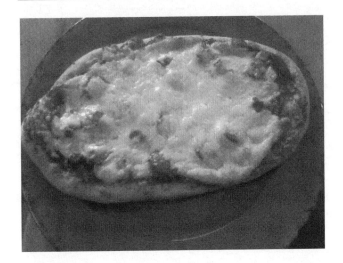

My pizza made with nomato sauce, ground beef and sliced up all natural beef franks that taste like smoked sausage.

It really is shocking how much this nomato sauce taste like tomato sauce!

*Warning- If you are salicylate sensitive, the ingredients in this recipe are considered moderate salicylates, eating many helpings of this could result in a reaction. (I learned this the hard way too!)

I have provided links to the different diets.

Salicylate Diet:

http://salicylatesensitivity.com/

Gluten Free Diet:

http://www.mayoclinic.org/healthy-living/nutrition-and-healthy-eating/in-depth/gluten-free-diet/art-20048530

Dairy Free Diet:

http://www.mayoclinic.org/diseases-conditions/lactose-intolerance/basics/definition/con-20027906

Elimination Diet:

http://www.fammed.wisc.edu/sites/default/files/webfm-uploads/documents/outreach/im/handout_elimination_diet_patient.pdf

Low Histamine Diet:

http://www.mastocytosis.ca/MSC%20HT%20Restricted%20Diet%20Nov2012.pdf

The Failsafe Diet:

http://www.failsafediet.com/

Another diet to consider is the Paleo Diet

http://thepaleodiet.com/

Chapter 16: Work

"Choose a job you love, and you will never have to work a day in your life."

Confusius

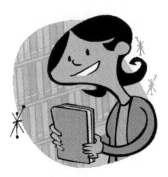

As the months marched on, it was all I could do to get up, go to work, come home, put my pajamas on, and go to bed. I loved my job, but I dreaded going there. At the time I didn't know why. I was a new hire at the local public library. It was a smooth transition into the new job, with the exception of an older lady who did not like me much. I went out of my way to be nice to this lady, but it just didn't seem to work. This just added stress to the days we worked together.

The job was fun and I enjoyed interacting with the public. I notice I felt better on my days off, but who doesn't, right? I would come home from work feeling horrible from head to toe and as red as a beet! A few times at work I would have to run to the bathroom and then wonder how I was ever going to get out of the bathroom. On a few occasions, my boss let me leave to go home, because I was not doing anyone any good stuck in the bathroom. I apologized profusely. I know she could see that I was ill.

As the weeks went on, my reactions at work became more and more severe. When I was first hired, I was healthy. I was a little tired from an infection, but a normal 40-year-old otherwise. My reactions started out as flushing and becoming very fatigued. My symptoms escalated to severe diarrhea, hives on my body and in my throat, and my hands and feet itching. These symptoms would take a few hours to kick in. As time went on, it took less and less time for the symptoms to start after I arrived at work. I was convinced that something at work was causing me these issues. This was also around the time I could not go into my house without having a reaction. I started to go into anaphylaxis after getting to work. It was like going to work was hurting me. I finally made a decision to quit. I was so upset because I loved the job, but my body would not cooperate with me. I would pre-medicate. I would take Benadryl while there. It just would not work. One time I had to leave early to go to the Immediate Care Center. I just could not keep it up physically. I was exhausted and figured that something in the building was causing it. Looking back, I am guessing that the books with book mold and a building that had a history of water leaks were to blame, along with the patrons who wore fragrances. Stress is also a mast cell degranulator, so having stressful days made things a lot worse.

Sara was a wonderful boss and I had great co-workers. I loved being part of the team. I miss those friendships. My time there was too short. I had no choice but to quit my job.

You know you have a good boss when they let you cry on their shoulder when you give them your resignation. Thank you, Sara, for the compassion you gave to me.

The only thing worse than quitting a job you love is not being able to go back for a visit.

Chapter 17: Disability

"Anyone who doesn't take truth seriously in small matters cannot be trusted in large ones either."

Albert Einstein

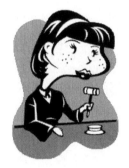

Unfortunately, even after quitting my job, my health continued to decline to the point of having anaphylaxis every few days. I was pretty much bed-ridden until later when I was put on mast cell stabilizers.

It was at this point that I applied for disability. I felt embarrassed to apply, like I was depending on the government or taking a handout. I was given a few nasty remarks from my "friends". Maybe that is why I felt a little funny about applying. The truth of the matter is they had opinions, but my friends quickly became unavailable to help me in any way. I started working when I was 13 years old. So I had all my credits needed to apply. I have been paying into this for years. I need it now, I should apply for the help, and it is my money.

Not surprisingly, I was denied; I heard that everyone gets denied the first few times. I hired a lawyer and did have to go to the hearing. I was completely honest answering the questions at the hearing. My lawyer said that I legally qualified, and the judge would have to throw out by entire testimony to deny me.

Several months later, I received a denial letter. It was based on the opinion of the judge that it couldn't be as bad as I had said. I was heartbroken that I had been truthful about everything and she just didn't believe me. Why did she bother to ask me questions if she was just going to say she didn't believe me? I told the truth in everything. Again, I think this is a situation where the truth sounds crazy and unbelievable.

Another reason for the denial was that I had anaphylaxis without having any allergies. Apparently, it is a concept people can't wrap their heads around. If someone would take the time to research mast cell issues BEFORE making life-changing decisions, they would have found out that with mast cell reactions you don't have to have IGE Allergies.

She also mentioned that if I could go out to eat, then I must be fine.

Now it seems that she was not asking me questions for the answers but asking me questions to find ways to trip me up. She had asked me if I was able to go out to eat. I answered a simple "yes". Don't answer a simple "yes". If I knew then what I know now, my answer would have been "On days that I am feeling excellent, I try to go out to eat. I have three places that are safe for me to eat. At these places I have looked up the ingredients in every food that I will eat. I have carefully chosen safe foods for me to eat. I will talk to the chef on occasion about my selection to ensure that the ingredients have not changed. Upon arriving at a location we always asked to be seated away from other people. We always ask to avoid an aisle seat. We only visit restaurants at off times when we know less people will be there. So yes, I can go out to eat, but when I do I must realize that I am putting my life in the hands of the waitress and the chef. I don't take this lightly, but at some point I try to find a little normalcy for myself and my family. I can't force everyone to eat at home for every meal". That is my answer -- that is what I should have said.

My lawyer has filed my last appeal. It has been almost 3 years since I applied. I stay home where I can control my environment. I cannot think of a place that would be safe for me to work. I was told at the disability hearing that I should be able to work in a sterile environment making computer chips. I can't help but laugh at this idea. I wish I was allowed to ask the judge a few questions...and if given another hearing, I just might. Are there companies that make computer chips in my area? Is there a place to sleep off the Benadryl that I will need to take after my coworker walks past with fragrance on? Do I get a nap time at this place? Do you understand that fragrance is not just perfume, but in fabric softeners, shampoos, conditioners, and lotion? Do you understand that I am missing the interactions with people? Do you realize I am missing being a valued member of a team? Do you realize I am missing being productive in a way that makes you feel good about a day's work? Do you understand the emotional toll that this has taken on me and my family? Do you know what it is like to feel worthless and then be told by a judge that they don't believe me? Do you understand that I have paid into this system for most of my life and by not taking the time to learn about mast cell reactions you are making an uneducated decision that will affect me the rest of my life; not only me, but my family? Oh and I have another question...do you know how lucky you are? If you get sick you can take an antibiotic without having to worry that the medicine might actually kill you...if you get dry skin you can just put lotion on, without wondering if it will cause a reaction. Do you know how lucky you are that you can go any place you want without calculating the risk involved? You can actually hug your kid without having a reaction?

A year before my hearing I was sent to a mandatory psychological evaluation. At this evaluation I was asked what I do for fun or what I do to enjoy myself. My response was that I was very ill, but on days that I felt well enough I would go outside and enjoy a sunny day.

At the hearing she asked me if I could go outside. My answer again was yes, because I can walk outside to the car or the mailbox without any problems. She asked me if I had problems with the heat and I said yes, the heat and humidity is problematic for me. My denial letter stated that, in her opinion, not only could I work, I could also work outside, because a year earlier I had made the comment that I like to go outside and enjoy the sunny day. When I went outside to enjoy the sunny day, I never sat in direct sunlight. I sat under our gazebo in the shade. Just because one enjoys a sunny day does not make them a sunbather! Since I mentioned enjoying a sunny day a year before, she used that, along with the fact that I could go outside, and concluded I could work outside. I find this obnoxious!

For the record, I can't be in direct sunlight. It burns my skin. I feel like a vampire most of the time. The judge never asked me if I could stand in direct sunlight, instead she asked if I could go outside and then she filled in the rest all on her own.

If I have learned anything from this experience it would be to never leave anything unsaid. If you are asked a question, answer it completely and thoroughly. If you have a symptom, don't neglect to mention it no matter how small.

Normally, when you think of a judge, you think of a person who is impartial. They don't have a personal interest in which side wins. However, in this case it is obvious that I was asked these questions in order to use the answers against me. Remember my experience if you have a disability hearing. I believe the judge is working to defend the State against the financial claim, which makes them biased.

Chapter 18: Food Diary

"Memories are the key not to the past, but to the future."

Corrie Ten Boom

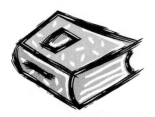 So let's talk about a food diary. It is called a food diary, but really it should be called a "I ate, I flushed, I had diarrhea, I threw up, I took my meds, I reacted diary". You want to record EVERYTHING, but we will just refer to it as a food diary.

You are going through all the trouble to figure out what you are reacting to. You HAVE to write it down and track your symptoms; it is too hard to try to remember what food bothered you last Monday, or was it Friday, no it was Tuesday...you get the point. Writing it down will prove to be so valuable.

You don't need to order a fancy food diary online. You can if that is the only way you will record stuff, but it is not necessary. My husband made one for me. I recorded the food I ate, the meds I took and any reactions during the day, including anaphylaxis, diarrhea, and nausea. I included days I went to work. Shoot, I even recorded when we had sex, because I knew I was allergic to my husband at this point and thought it might be a good idea to track it.

The idea is to look for a pattern. I had a regular sized piece of paper for every day. Interestingly enough I started taping mine to the bedroom wall. Several months into this I had an entire wall covered with papers. I did kind of feel like a mad professor because I would sit on the bed and just stare, looking for some kind of pattern. Honestly, I never found it, because I have a salicylate sensitivity. Salicylates are in so many foods, that you easily consume them in every meal. Salicylates stack and this makes them very hard to track. So did I waste my time with the food diary? Absolutely NOT- Once I suspected the salicylate issues, looking at the food diary confirmed my suspicions! It was there, it was just hidden so well that it would have been impossible to see without suspicions. I have also been able to use my food diary for my disability claim. It had all the dates of my reactions and the severity of them. I can honestly say on June 4, 2012 I had diarrhea three times! How is that for record keeping!

What better way to keep all of your discoveries than a notebook? I'm talking about the old fashion pen and paper here! Now my husband uses the computer for notes but I find a notebook can travel with you. It is like flat Stanley, it can go with you to your appointments, and meetings. When I come across something that I think may be important I write it in my notebook, I think I am on notebook number three. I file them in a filing cabinet so that I can go back and look things up. If you think you are reacting to something, make a note about it. Keep good records. Between the food diary and note taking you will start to see potential problems.

Chapter 19: Emergency Notebooks, Emergency Situations

"Intellectuals solve problems, geniuses prevent them."

Albert Einstein

A friend told me to make an Emergency Notebook. She told me this folder/notebook would be able to "talk" for me in the event that I could not. So, I want to pass this information on. This is very useful if you are a "shocker" and require ER visits. A "shocker" is some-one who reacts and goes into anaphylaxis. If you are not a shocker you may be called a "leaker". This is someone who constantly has symptoms, or leaks symptoms. Being a shocker helps identify your triggers faster. Leaking symptoms constantly makes iden-tifying triggers harder. There is no winner here, it is not better to be a leaker or a shocker.

Thankfully, I have never been alone during one of these episodes that required emergency help. However, I always take my Emergency folder along for the nurses and/or doctors to look at. (They actually do!)

I recommend writing ANAPHYLAXIC SHOCKING DISORDER-instead of MASTOCYTOSIS or MCAS. The reason being, an EMT knows what and how to treat ana-phylaxis, but may never have heard of Mastocytosis or MCAS. This could waste time if he or she is afraid to treat you. You should definitely include the Mastocytosis Emer-gency Protocol. They can read about it after they treat you for anaphylaxis!

I think this notebook is the first line of defense in getting the doctors and nurses to listen to you, to understand this is a chronic condition, not just an isolated situation or a panic attack. Most doctors don't like to be told how to treat you. This folder does that without you saying a word. I think it is important to make your specialist's information available. That is why I carry the specialist's card so she can be contacted, if needed.

At my last ER visit the nurses wanted a list of the medicines I am currently taking, and suggested I add that to the folder, so I did! I also keep a list of my known allergies.

One of the most important pieces I have in my folder is a signed paper from the specialist requesting certain tests to be performed. Doctors will usually honor your specialist requests. Now, if you think about it, having your specialist ask for certain tests and sign the paperwork is kind of like having your specialist say "This is my patient and he or she will most likely be having an allergic reaction that can lead to anaphylaxis. When this happens, please run these tests for me." This will help with getting the doctor to listen to you, because your specialist is involved in the situation.

I also have a few pictures of me swollen, which confirm to whoever looks at the folder that indeed I do have allergic reactions. I don't get these pictures out, I just have them hanging on one of the three rings in the notebook. It is hard to argue with a picture. Now don't carry 14 shots of a swollen face. 1 or 2 will be plenty; the nurses don't have time to look at more than 1 or 2 pictures. It wouldn't hurt to have a normal head shot along with the 1 or 2 swollen pictures. This makes it easier to tell if you are swollen at that moment. Remember, these nurses and doctors don't know what you normally look like. If you don't have visual swelling, then don't worry about the pictures.

Understand that the ER doctor has to start at square one when you arrive without any information about your disorder. Starting from square one makes it very easy for you to get the old panic attack diagnosis, because, let's face it, sometimes that is what it looks like. We know differently, but they don't.

Doctors are trained to look for horses, not zebras, so take that folder in and say... "Look, I am a zebra", long before they have a chance to call you a horse.

I also think trying to remain as calm as possible can only help. I know this is extremely stressful and scary but going to the ER in a panic looks like panic!

By taking an hour or so to prepare an emergency notebook, you are saving yourself the trouble of once again trying to explain, in a Benadryl stupor, what mast cells are and how you think you should be treated. I have made one for each vehicle and one for the house in the event of a 911 call. This gives me peace of mind and the ability to remain as calm as possible.

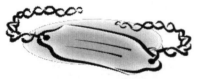 Another useful tool to consider is a medical ID bracelet. This informs first responders of your allergies and needs in the event of an emergency situation if you are alone or you don't have your emergency folder with you. Mine simply states my name, Aspirin and food allergies, EPI.

Also, medical personnel are trained to look for these medical ID's when you arrive at the ER. Wearing a bracelet that indicates that you need EPI or have allergies will be noted. There is a pretty good chance that you won't be labelled as a person with anxiety, but a person with a chronic condition that frequently requires medical intervention. I wear my bracelet 24/7; I never take it off. That way it will be there when I need it.

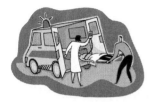
Another useful tool in an emergency situation is a security system. Most security systems now have fire, police and emergency buttons, to get help to your house. The security system we use is cellular and does not need a home phone line, which is good if you don't have a home phone. The one we installed came with a medical pendant. Now, I kind of snicker at the idea of me wearing a medical pendant because of that silly "I have fallen and can't get up commercial." However, if I am alone and need emergency help, it is only a button away. My husband informed me I should wear it during a bad week. I agreed I would! Notice he said bad week. He knows if I have a bad trigger, I will be having a bad week. We think of it as insurance. You hope you never need it, but when you do you are glad you have it. Plus the system provides security.

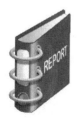
I also recommend using a three ring binder to hold lab results. I have always asked for a copy of the lab results so that I have them at hand for myself or a doctor. They are your results so you have a right to them. I think it is good to have a copy. Looking back over the lab results I can tell that the mast cell stabilizers made a difference, just in my CBC!

One of the hardest parts of Mast Cell Disorder is how unpredictable it is. The feeling of having no control over the situation is so stressful. By making the folder, wearing a medical bracelet and having a system in place that can get me medical attention at the push of a button; I have taken back a little control. I have a little peace of mind knowing that if I can't speak for myself, they will.

I have included some pictures for your enjoyment!

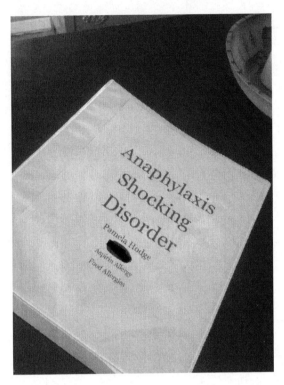

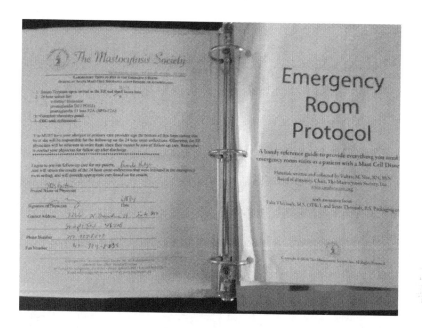

This is the important paper where your specialist "informs" the E.R. doctor that you are their patient and that most likely you will be needing emergency treatment and, in that event, to please run certain test. Again, this will involve your specialist in your treatment at the E.R. Also make sure your specialist's phone number is readily available. The emergency room protocol provides the nurses and doctors with a list of medications to avoid and medications that are usually safe to administer.

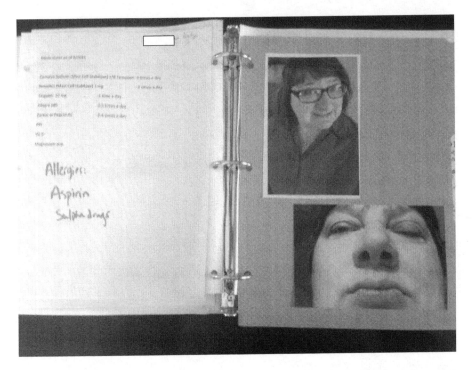

This is a list of the drugs that I take on a daily basis and my allergies. I have also included a glamour shot of regular me and nasty masty me.

You can find the Emergency Room Protocol at http://www.tmsforacure.org/documents/ER_Protocol.pdf

You are welcome!! ☺

Chapter 20: Broken Friendships

"Loneliness is never more cruel than when it is felt in close propinquity with someone who has ceased to communicate."

Germaine Greer

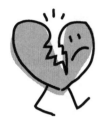 I would like to be able to say that my life is back to the way it was before all this started, that things haven't changed that much -- but that's not the truth. In fact, this is one of reasons I decided to write this book. The isolation and loneliness that I have felt over the last few years has been so hard to deal with. I am hoping someone will read this book and understand their friend or relative better. I am hoping that instead of jumping to conclusions, they will pause and consider doing research and being the support system that any ill person needs.

People who have Mast Cell disorders are not crazy. They are not having panic attacks. They are having real reactions to triggers. It is not something they caused. It is not something they can control, nor can the timing of their symptoms be controlled. Diagnosis can take several years and several doctors. I was told by my friend that I went from doctor to doctor trying to find out what is wrong. Anyone with an unknown chronic illness will go from specialist to specialist and even be misdiagnosed several times before finding the right doctor who can make the correct diagnosis. This is an extremely rare disorder, therefore it is usually not considered by specialists unless they specialize in mast cell issues or have knowledge of it.

The dust has settled, but in the storm I lost a few friends. You think your friends will weather whatever comes, but I guess that doesn't always happen. My friends, who I have known for years, have said some terribly hurtful things -- things that are hard to forgive and likely never to be forgotten. I have been laughed at, criticized, and ignored. I have been accused of being a hypochondriac and bi-polar, all this from my "friends", who to this day show no remorse or concern. One told me flat out that they don't believe me. They don't have to believe me. I am not a doctor; I did not do the diagnosing. I don't want belief anyway; I am still in disbelief myself.

I wanted a little compassion and understanding. I guess as humans we expect to get from others what we are willing to give. I have always been willing to treat others with respect and I guess I am wrong to just expect it.

My advice from experience: don't talk about your crisis to anyone who doesn't really want to help. Also don't talk about your crisis to anyone who is dealing with their own crisis. It can be perceived as insensitive. I learned this from experience. I was told I was insensitive and uncaring because I spoke about my illness when she was dealing with her own crisis. Looking back, I can see how I was dealing with my situation, while she was dealing with her situation. I am, however, saddened to be accused of not caring. That is the farthest thing from the truth. Perhaps that was a reflection of her feelings. They certainly were not mine.

I think I made the mistake of sharing too much in the beginning. With this disease, things change from hour to hour. You can go from being fine to having anaphylaxis in just minutes. I guess when this happens it looks made up or unbelievable.

I am not going to sit here and say that I never looked or acted crazy. My whole situation was out of control. I was in fight or flight mode most of the time for many months.

This happens when you go into anaphylaxis; there is a feeling of impending doom. If you google anaphylaxis, you will find that is actually a symptom of it. There is an element of anxiety here. Anaphylaxis is not just swelling of the throat. There is a lot happening in the body. Heart rate and BP spike, because the blood vessels start dilating and once they dilate so far the heart rate and BP plummet. There is also lots of diarrhea and vomiting (thankfully, I don't vomit that much). All this mixed with the high doses of antihistamines; I was probably all over the place. I have talked with my specialist about how this has affected my friendships. He told me, and wanted me to tell my friends, that mast cells can affect brain function. He said cognitive function and behavior can be affected. But this does not make me crazy or bi- polar. It just means I was sick and needed the proper treatment. I don't quite understand how or why my friends questioned the diagnosis I was given.

As many of you know, one of the hardest parts of this illness is the rejection we feel when people don't believe us. Surviving from day to day can be extremely hard, but watching people walk away is painful. I was accused of having a mental illness by my best friend; she refused to listen to the specialist, refused to see the improvement when I went on mast cell stabilizers and even refused to acknowledge anything to do with "my illness." To her, I made the whole thing up. Why would anyone make up an illness that requires you to give up so much of your life?

Have you ever wondered how someone just walks away when you need them the most? The answer I have gotten for that question is that their true colors are showing and I should be glad to finally see them clearly. I agree with whoever told me this, but don't you wonder how a person lives with themselves when they very clearly made a mistake and refuse to acknowledge it? Do they just pretend every day that they were right to do and say those things? Do they have a conscience?

If you have friends who hang in there with you and are there supporting you, know you are blessed and hold tight to those friends. They are the ones willing to learn and understand. There are going to be people who walk away and that is heart-breaking and at times unbelievable, but, in reality, do you want someone in your life who doesn't care enough to understand or to even try to educate themselves on the disease? Will it be easy? No. By all means, being rejected and doing it gracefully is very hard work.

To you, my oldest friend, it occurred to me that I never have taken the opportunity to respond to your letter. The one indicating that you didn't believe me, that I am just playing the victim, and that this is just another illness in the long list since you have known me. Don't worry, I will not post it again, as that made you angry and you haven't spoken to me since. The letter was so hurtful that I needed some advice from others in my situation about how to handle it. I think that I should take this opportunity to respond to your comments, not only for me, but for every person who has this disease and has been in this situation.

So here is my response: I am sorry that you don't believe me about this illness, but that doesn't make me crazy. Besides, you were my "best" friend... shouldn't you still love and support me even if I did have a mental illness? I didn't know there was a stipulation on our friendship.

Come to think of it, you have had a few health issues of your own. I really never witnessed your ailment. Are you sure you needed that surgery? You experienced the symptoms and dealt with them many years. Just because I didn't see them doesn't mean they didn't happen, does it?

Guess what, I believed you and never, ever questioned that you had something serious that needed treatment. I never accused you of making it up and playing a victim. So why is it you don't believe me? Why is it you don't believe the allergist/immunologist who has been practicing medicine for over 30 years?

You had mentioned that I change doctors constantly and stories just as often. Yes, it was so exhausting finding a doctor who finally figured it out. You are right; I have been to a long list of them. Why is that a problem for you exactly? I was referred to an endocrinologist and a rheumatologist by my regular doctor because of test results. I did go to two different rheumatologists, but I remember that you switched doctors for similar reasons when you were not satisfied with the care you received. I saw my allergist/immunologist for over two years until he sent me to a different allergist/immunologist that specializes in aspirin allergy. I have been seeing her over a year. Now if anyone is sorry that it takes years to diagnose mast cell disease, it is me and countless others who suffer from a rare condition. Countless symptoms followed by countless doctors. The doctor finally figured it out. After all those years, I really wish you would have been happy for me, not telling me to get "REAL" help. Believe me, I have been so close to feeling crazy by dealing with this, but I can honestly tell you now that on the right medications, I am becoming more and more like my old self.

Regarding the comment about changing stories, there were several working theories by various doctors before they ruled out everything else. This is a common experience for people with a rare condition. They are commonly misdiagnosed for years before receiving the correct diagnosis.

About the day we were supposed to eat out, but I got upset and you didn't know why - I would like to explain why I was upset. We had planned on meeting at 1 p.m. I had been stuck in the house for a while and I was looking forward to having lunch with you. Cromolyn (mast cell stabilizer) is a medicine I have to drink four times a day. Every dose must be timed at least 2 hours after eating. Then I have to wait another 30 minutes before eating. It has to be absorbed through the stomach without food. I had timed it out that day, so that at 1 p.m. I could eat lunch with you.

You called and said you were done early and asked if we could we eat much earlier than planned. I said "no, I can't eat now". I tried to meet you in the middle by asking if noon would work, do you remember? You never asked why, but insisted that we eat earlier. Apparently, you called the third party and she called me and insisted that you both were meeting earlier, even though I told her I couldn't. So when I brought Beth and dropped her off, you both were already eating and enjoying your lunch. Yes, I was upset and angry that you were eating without me, that you couldn't wait and hour or so. What I needed didn't matter at all to either of you. Can you honestly say this wouldn't upset you?

You also accused me of odd behavior because I went to an eye doctor and held vials of allergens while he walked around me. Again, I would have been more than happy to explain that if given the chance. I went to a doctor who practiced NAET which stands for Nambudripad's Allergy Elimination Technique. This is a holistic approach to eliminating allergies. Yes, he was an eye doctor, but he also specialized in NAET. He specialized in two things. I was desperate to find answers and have read that NAET really helps some people. Even if you have never heard of it, and thought it made me look a little looney, that doesn't mean it isn't effective for some, it just means you have never heard of it. I was hoping it would help me. Maybe it did, maybe it didn't. Why would this matter to you?

You mentioned that I had gotten worse over the past few years and the fun Pam is gone. I can't agree with you more on this. I had gotten worse, a lot worse. I became worse yet after you stopped speaking to me. It has been a rough 3 years. Yes, the fun Pam was hard to find. I spent many weeks in bed. I was literally in bed, too sick to get up except to go poo or vomit. You have to give me a little leeway here; I don't know too many people who are fun under those circumstances.

You said if I were really sick with all that I claim to have had I would be in the hospital or worse. I have been in the hospital - many times. Again, just because you don't know about a situation doesn't make it any less true.

Now I have something to ask you. Why would you call me up after ignoring me for 6 plus months to tell me that Mr. Smith (name changed) had tests and the results are not good and inform me-that is what real illness looks like? Really? After ignoring me and not having a clue what I was going through just to survive from day to day, you have the nerve to call me up and try to educate me on what true illness is. Let me educate you a little - mast cell disorders can be life threatening at any given moment if you go into anaphylaxis or if you have organ or blood involvement. There is no cure. There is only medicine to try to control the symptoms. Believe me - I know what real illness is. I know how it has taken my world and turned it upside down. There are others that are sick and just hanging on, but that doesn't give you the right to call me up and try to convince me that I'm not "really" ill and compare me to others. I was far too gracious to you that day. I should have put you in your place. Your attitude was rude, condescending and completely unnecessary.

The bottom line is I have felt for the past three years, when I needed a friend the most, you were avoiding me. I have had a real sense of loss, and every once in a while something will remind me of you and that loss is still there. But I have accepted the situation and moved on. I am feeling a bit foolish because I have always thought of you like family -- like no matter what, we could depend on each other. Can you at all step into my shoes here and, just for a moment, feel the disappointment I have felt? I ask that, when in reality, I don't think you can. I really don't think that you are capable of feeling empathy for people.

I believe there has been a lot of miscommunication, or more accurately, no communication. I think you made your mind up and that was that.

Your opinion should have never been presented as fact to anyone, ever. How could you do that? One, is it just a horrible thing to do and two, what will you do if you're wrong. You either have to keep pretending you were right or you have to admit you were wrong and I don't think you can do that. No one can be right about everything 100% of the time. We all make mistakes, most of which can be remedied, but by far the biggest mistake is not admitting them.

I think it is sad and a waste of a 15-year friendship, because any one of those times I have been rushed to the ER, you should have been there beside me, holding my hand assuring me everything would be okay.

I am truly sorry you could not see the truth. I am saddened that, even if you have realized the truth, you haven't apologized and tried to make it right with me. The fact that our friendship wasn't worth an apology, I think, is the saddest part of all. That fact says a lot about you and makes me see our friendship from a different perspective. A perspective that is clearer and more honest.

I am sure, in your mind, you have a good reason for your actions, but for the record I would have been there for you... holding your hand.

"Love me or hate me both are in my favor...If you love me I'll always be in your heart...If you hate me I will always be in your mind."

William Shakespeare

"A FRIEND is one who walks in when others walk out."

Jerome Cummings

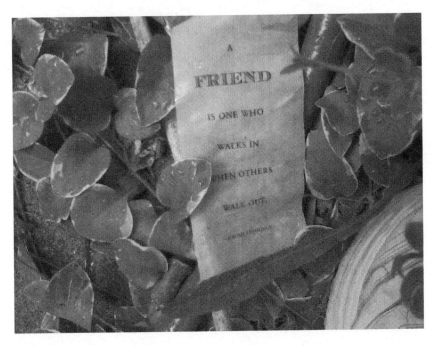

I found this one morning outside in my yard. It was reassurance of what friendship looks like. I believe it was sent to me at the time I needed to see it the most. It was a little morning miracle.

Chapter 21: Grief and Depression

"Heavy hearts, like heavy clouds in the sky, are best relieved by the letting of a little water."

Christopher Morley

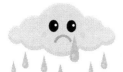 Having a chronic illness can result in grief. Having crazy mast cells can result in depression.

I have grieved the loss of a lot in the past three years - my old life, my job, my freedom and even the loss of foods. It is sad to watch people eat knowing you can't touch it. That hits on an emotion that is hard to express.

I have learned a little about the grieving process itself. There are 5 steps.

Denial and Isolation- this is a coping mechanism that helps us to deal with the immediate shock of a situation.

Anger-we can be angry at everyone or no one.

Bargaining-If only we had done something different or if I change something the outcome will be different.

Depression-We feel sad and may have a lot of regret.

Acceptance-Acceptance of the situation can take a long time. In the case of chronic illness it is easier when you finally get to the acceptance stage. You finally realize there is nothing to do to fix it, or change it. You just simply accept it. Sadness is finally replaced by little glimpses of thankfulness and happiness. This is a very slow process. Each time the mast cells show me they are in charge, I tend to slide back into step 4-depression. I think it is a process that never really will be completed.

Depression for me is different than grief. Now it is a symptom of something going on. I often wonder if the 10+ years I took antidepressants were actually my mast cells firing away. I will never know. What I do know...in 12 hours without Cromolyn or the right dose of Cromolyn I can spiral down into the deep depths of despair. I can be happy as a lark and then 12 hours later be a total mess. My cognitive function is totally lacking and decision making is next to impossible. It is as if I am a robot and I need someone to tell me what to do and when. I am angry and feeling overwhelmed with sadness. I watched that happen yesterday, more horrifying - my husband watched that happen!

After a big trigger I do become depressed for a few days, it is like clockwork. It helps with the depression to know the reason and to know it is going to be temporary. Usually within three days or so I feel less sad and start to laugh at myself again. Believe me, during those few days after a trigger, nothing is funny. I feel sad, depressed and overwhelmed. Pretty much how I felt for months when all of this started and I was triggering every day or having anaphylaxis several times a week. Those were some rough months.

I posted a saying the other day on the group wall that hit a nerve. It said "The bravest thing I have ever done was continuing my life when I wanted to die." Being completely honest here, yes, I hate to admit it, there was a time when I was that low. I think I hit rock bottom. I was triggering every day, I felt betrayed by my friends, and I was in a deep depression. I didn't really care what happened to me. I remember trying so hard to just feel happiness, some thread of happiness, but I didn't feel anything, just overwhelming sadness. I didn't care if I lived or died, but I did care about my husband and kids, I did care how they would feel.

I truly believe that the Cromolyn is what has helped with my depression. I believe it is helping by controlling the mast cells. If I skip a dose, I will be depressed the next day. I never do that on purpose, but some days I will forget to take it at a certain time and it throws off my whole schedule.

I was reading the other day that depression is not a symptom of mast cell issues but just part of it. In other words, it doesn't happen because our lives suck and we are sad, but it happens as part of the chemical processes going on in our brain. If you are having depression, don't feel bad or embarrassed about it. It may just be part of the disease. You may just need to be on the right mast cell stabilizers or medications to get that under control. If you hit rock bottom, know that you are not alone; others have been there and made their way out. It is a sad and lonely place, but you really are never alone, you just feel that way. It also helps to remember that the mast cells are messing with reality and that once you get the disease under control your depression will lessen or go away.

When I am having a really bad day, I just have to remember how far I have come. At one point I realized how very important the small things in life are. If the bad times have taught me anything, it is to stop and slow down and really enjoy every good moment. How could we ever know what the good moments are if we had nothing to compare them to? I try to find the humor and beauty in every day. I try to live in the moment, to savor the good times and to laugh as much as I can, because the sound of laughter is healing to everyone around us.

The wallpaper on my phone has two words - "Be Happy". These words used to be a goal, now they are a reminder, a reminder of the many things I have to be happy about.

"Affliction comes to us, not to make us sad but sober; not to make us sorry but wise."
- H. G. Wells

"Our real blessings often appear to us in the shape of pains, losses and disappointments; but let us have patience and we soon shall see them in their proper figures."

Joseph Addison

I have seen several times just in the last few years that bad things are going to happen. The amazing thing is I have seen good come out of the bad things.

One Saturday I awoke with that jiggly feeling and my heart racing. So knowing that I am having a histamine dump or a reaction, I grab a Benadryl and some water to chug it down, barely even opening an eye in the process. I keep one Benadryl nearby for these kinds of mornings. They are happening more and more and I need to figure that out. As you can imagine, when you take a Benadryl in the early morning, you might tend to sleep in. On this particular morning, my husband came in the bedroom and asked if I was awake yet? I was like "well my head is a wake, but the rest of me is sleeping, why?" We have a mess downstairs and I need your help. Uh oh, those are not good words. So, in my early morning Benadryl Stupor, I got dressed and headed down the stairs to a mess that I knew was too big for Dan to handle alone. I figured the dogs had eaten another dog bed or dragged the contents of someone's underwear drawer out to the back-yard...again. I am guessing the neighbors tend to laugh every time there is a bra on the back lawn. The dogs really hate to be left alone!

Once I'm downstairs Dan points me in the right direction. He said it was in the fridge. Now I thought "how bad could that be??" Something spilled in the fridge? That is not cool but can be wiped up and I can be snoozing again in no time! No, he said, not a spill, something froze and blew up. It turns out our Oberweis chocolate milk in the glass jar froze in the refrigerator then blew up like a little liquid chocolate bomb. It looked like a crime scene! Every inch of the refrigerator was chocolate! My jaw dropped, now that IS a big mess! Dan had already started the cleaning process when he realized he needed backup. I think I needed some backup too! Back up the stairs to my bed!

We had owned this fridge less than one year, it is a reminder of my last huge trigger, Epi and ER visit. I knew we were coming up to the year anniversary. Yes, you start thinking in terms of 'it has been x amount of time since my last Epi.' Or call it my Epi anniversary! Funny how life can change and we can enjoy some of the smallest accomplishments.

I always get nervous when purchasing new appliances. You know, you slap down a lot of money and then you are stuck using the appliance for several years. It is hard to pick out an appliance in a few hours that you will be happy with for years to come. I mean really - that is a hard thing to do. How do you know until you use the thing for a few months? We try to spend a little more and use them longer. My husband always says you get what you pay for. In this particular case, we had decided to get a very well known "fancy" brand that was a floor model. We figured that they were discounting the fridge because it was a floor model and they weren't selling that brand anymore, so we would be getting the Cadillac of fridges for the price of a regular model. We were paying a bit more than we should on the floor model but since it was a Cadillac, we thought it was the best thing to do. It looked great, there were a few scratches on it but that can easily be covered with a magnet. Once we got it home we realized how small it was compared to the one we had before. But it's a Cadillac! After all, it is a really great fridge and we have a freezer in the garage for over flow. So we were happy with our purchase. We went ahead and ordered the extended warranty. It has all the fancy temps, buttons, bells and whistles. I like all those things but in my mind I just figure that it is something that will go out and need repaired down the road.

Being close to the year anniversary date, I have come to regret our decision on the small Cadillac. It is too small. I want some room in the freezer to freeze all my meat before the histamines start to grow. I know - first world problem. So now that it has been only less than a year and it is already having temperature issues, I am really disappointed. We have thrown away tons of veggies that have frozen over the last few months and now this. Something is not right on our new fridge. I am cleaning milk off of every surface in there and ranting and raving about calling them to come out to fix it when it isn't even a year old. Dan is just being calm as usual. I wanted to call and complain to someone right then and there and he said "Lets clean first. Then we will find the paper work and call."

Being grumpy, tired and smelling like milk was not my idea of a nice Saturday morning. I even said out loud "this is not my idea of a good morning." We started high and worked our way down. Of course, the milk was on the top shelf. We got down to the drawers and could not figure out how in the world to remove them. We couldn't take the drawer out, let alone the drawer compartment. The milk was in the drawers, running down behind the compartment, and no matter what we tried that drawer was not coming out.

So we got the phone and called customer service. We explained our dilemma and the nice lady on the phone needed the model and serial number. So after reading through 27 numbers, she asked if we were John Smith? (Name changed) What? No...that is not the correct name! Here, let's go over the 27 numbers again while we are dripping in chocolate milk as it drips onto the floor. I was really trying to have a good attitude here. Again, she says yes this refrigerator is registered to a John Smith. Oh my goodness - now I am really steamed. We have purchased a used refrigerator. I don't care if it is a Cadillac. It is used and returned, most likely because it has problems. So, I'm snorting and ranting and Dan is STILL calm. She continues to tell us how to remove the drawer compartment...the drawer does not come out of the compartment. My husband has a master's degree and it still took us ten minutes to figure it out even after she gave us the instructions. I am guessing you need a course in drawer removal to be proficient at it. So, as you can imagine, I am not liking this fridge...at all.

We continued to clean, but I am still on my rant. I tell him that it was not right to sell us a used fridge and not tell us. I told him I want a new fridge without problems and it needs to be bigger. He agreed that it wasn't right but he wasn't sure what the store would do to make it right, so I didn't get my hopes up too much. He thought they would probably just repair it and that would be it.

It took us all of two hours to get the whole mess cleaned up. We decided to go to the store and see what they would do, if anything. We went upstairs to get our paperwork together.

We definitely needed proof from the company that the refrigerator was registered in someone else's name. So we called the company and asked them with fingers crossed to please send us an email indicating that information and to please make sure it had the dates.

Thankfully the company agreed and sent it right over. After reading the information, it appeared that the fridge was originally purchased 6 years earlier...Dan was shocked and thought that couldn't be right. So we went on the hunt to find the manufacturing date located somewhere on the fridge. We found it!! It turns out that it was in fact over 6 years old! We had paid over a thousand dollars for a 6 year old fridge. At this point I burst out laughing because there is no way the store could get around fixing this!

Thankfully, the manager was a delight and he was very apologetic and he even thanked us for having a sense of humor...but really how was this not so strange that you couldn't laugh at it?! We got our bigger, new fridge the following week.

Looking back, I realize that if that chocolate milk had never exploded, we would still be using our soon to be 7 year old fridge that has lots of problems.

I have always been a person who believes that all things happen for a reason. I believe God works in all things. Romans 8:28: "And we know that God causes all things to work together for good to those who love God, to those who are called according to His purpose."

I can look back over the past several years and see several things that turned out much better than it looked in the beginning. The great flood helped us to locate the mold in the air duct system. The invasion of the voles led us to the leaky window. The loss and loneliness I felt when my friends decided I was crazy led me to start the My Crazy Life With Mast Cell Disorder group and to write this book. I have gotten several messages from people thanking me for the support and the group. Telling me it has made a difference in their lives. So I believe good has come from a bad situation. I lost two friends but gained countless more.

My mother has told me on several occasions that the reason I got this illness is because I am meant to help others. I quickly replied I would have helped them without being this sick...but really, would I? How would I have understood, if it wasn't for being in the same position. How would I have gotten it, without getting it?

"I see possibilities in everything. For everything that's taken away, something of greater value has been given."

Michael J. Fox

Chapter 23: Cognitive Dysfunction & Humor

"I have seen what a laugh can do. It can transform almost unbearable tears into something bearable, even hopeful."
Bob Hope

They say laughter is the best medicine. I do agree laughter helps in most situations. It is good to laugh at yourself, and it is good to laugh at yourself with others. There were some days, not so many now, where my brain just would not find the right words. Finding a word to complete a sentence was actually a task. Now, honestly, it is a very scary feeling being unable to access the language part of your brain. I would always come up with a word when this happened, but it was usually the wrong word. I would get these hilarious looks from my family...what in the heck are you trying to say? At first, I am sure they were concerned as I was, but over time it just became kind of funny to see what was going to come flying out of my mouth. Now, in my defense, I would always get close-well, sort of. Usually my words would come out starting with the same letter. "Do you want to have hangers for dinner?!" Short pause...wrong word. "I mean "hamburgers"?" Lots of giggling going on and me rolling my eyes, because once again I have been slapped with the stupid stick! Sometimes it took me so long to come up with the word we finally turned it into a game and called it "What is Pam trying to say?" Usually this was quite fun unless I was in a bad mood and I felt like my family was laughing at me, instead of with me. The rule of thumb is to remember they are not laughing at me, but with me.

Even now, after being stable for a while, after a big trigger I will get this weird inability to say words. I will usually say a sentence and then be surprised that I said something so stupid. It is like my brain and my mouth is not connected. Is it funny? Yes, actually laughing at yourself gets you over the feeling of stupid really fast. The family is used to this new way of communicating. It is actually a clue for me when I start coming up with words that don't fit the context or words that don't make sense that I am reacting to something. Who knew words could be so hard??

I'm still laughing about something I did last week. After having a reaction last week at the grocery store, I drove home starting to feel that weak, limp feeling. Thinking, "Wow, I need a nap now." I found myself trying to open my front door with the key fob to my car! Who does this? I was actually pushing the button! Bethany standing there saying "Uh, mom, that isn't going to work!" By the time she said it, I had figured that out! At least I was pushing the "unlock" button.

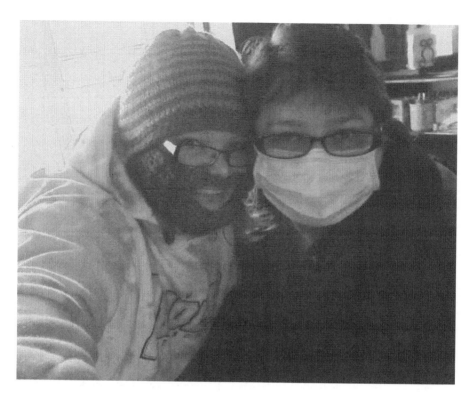

Pam & Beth: The Masked Duo!

Chapter 24: Swellings and Tellings

"People are like stained-glass windows. They sparkle and shine when the sun is out, but when the darkness sets in, their true beauty is revealed only if there is a light from within."

Elisabeth Kubler-Ross

Waking up swollen and looking like a different person can be humorous! It really is all in the attitude. I usually just try to laugh it off. I'm not going to lie, sometimes it is hard not looking like the person you were yesterday. But the swelling does eventually go away.

I recently took some swollen "glamour shots" of myself to give to the specialist. The nurse was amazed; she said she had never heard of angioedema before this job. She commented how the pictures all looked different from each other and none of them looked like me at all! I laughed and said "I know, crazy huh". Seems there is never a dull moment at our house. I have yet to understand most of the swelling. On days I think I will be swollen from being exposed to something, I'm not too swollen, but then some days I will wake up and think what in the world happened last night! Seems there is no rhyme or reason. This brings me to a frank discussion that was a little hard to accept from the doctor a few weeks ago. I gave her the pictures and we discussed different triggers and she told me that there are going to be cases where nothing is going to cause it. The mast cells are just going to get angry and act. Now intellectually I know this can happen, but on an emotional level, this is hard stuff to accept. This is admitting that in a lot of the circumstances I have no control. Having no control is upsetting in any circumstance.

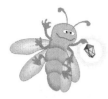 Like my specialist warned me, there was one evening in particular that I recall that really upset me because I went into anaphylaxis and I have no idea what caused it. Usually I can at least point to something and say it was this, whether it was or not. That usually makes me feel a little better about the situation. Remember, giving up all control in a situation is very hard! On this particular evening, I had eaten a banana a few hours before. I did notice a slight reaction but nothing to be too concerned over. I was sitting in the living room and had decided to go sit on the porch and call my mom. It was humid but not overly hot and a bit hazy that day, but it was around 7 P.M. so the heat of the day was over. I was just chatting away when suddenly I felt like I was choking on my own spit. Like I had sucked something into my windpipe. I started coughing, trying to get "it" up. My mom, who was on the phone, asked if I had swallowed a bug. Well, that is completely possible because it felt like I did! I told her to hold on a second while I tried to dislodge this bug! So after several attempts to get rid of this critter that has flown into my mouth and down my throat into my lungs all without me noticing it, I decided to go back into the house.

So, sitting in the living room, I was still uncomfortable with the feeling that I needed to cough it up. It was at this point that my throat started to feel tight. I realized that I had not taken any of my evening meds. I was only a half hour late on one, though. I told my mom I needed to hang up and take some medicine. So I start taking those -- Allegra, Zantac, Ketotifen and Singulair. I know that those are not emergency medicines but I hadn't deemed this an emergency yet. After all my meds were in, my throat was still swelling and I officially decided this was not stopping...so I added a Benadryl to my drug cocktail. I gave it a few minutes but I was still escalating, so I take a second Benadryl.

This is when I started to get anxious, because I knew the only thing left to help is the Epi Pen. So was the anxiety because of the situation or was it a chemical response? Most likely a little of both. I had Bethany call Dan and find out if he was still at the store or if he was almost home. I knew if I used the Epi Pen, I would need to go to the hospital and I didn't want to put Beth in the position to get me there. I can always hit the panic button on the alarm system and get an ambulance, but that is very costly. So, yes, I had all these thoughts flying around my head and, once again, the feeling of impending doom. So I gave myself a pep talk. It went something like this...You are fine. If you are not, you have your Epi on hand to help you. You can have emergency services here in a few minutes and they can help you. Bethany is here, so you are not alone. Dan is on his way, so just take some deep breaths. (Ha look I'm talking to myself...maybe I am a little crazy after all!) Whatever it takes to stay calm and let the medicine work.

So I narrowly made it out of that incident without using the Epi Pen. It was close and the rest of the evening I spent in the bathroom and bed, taking additional Benadryl as soon as I could.

Some would say I should have Epi-ed. Yes, I agree. Looking back, I should have. It is ALWAYS so much easier looking back at the situations to know what I should have done. I was also in a little bit of denial, because to me there was no obvious trigger.

I tell everyone else to err on the side of caution. I would never suggest "waiting it out a few minutes". So don't read this and think this is what you should do. You have to create a plan with your doctor and follow it. Only you know how your body will react. Throat swelling is dangerous. I think there is a learning curve. I have dealt with my throat swelling so much that I may be a bit callused to the danger of it all. I do have a plan in place. I do follow it. For me, I give the Benadryl a few minutes to work. If they don't, I move on to Epi.

A few days after this mystery trigger I worked up the courage to go to the fair. It happens once a year and I wanted to go. I was very cautious and did what I could to be safe. Again, in hindsight, I am wondering if that was the brightest thing to do. I mean, if you think about it, the fair is full of people, animals and smells. It actually could have been very dangerous, but I was prepared in the event of an emergency. I did have to take a Benadryl, but overall I think I did well for me.

I went to a family reunion recently. I think I may have been the first to leave, but I was happy that I was able to go and see the family. Can't leave the Bat Cave for too long! I ate only safe foods, had a good time and left in good shape. I think Dan helped me stay on track by going and making my plate. He knows what I can eat and this helped me avoid temptation that could have landed me in the hospital. I know the foods that are big no-no's for me are tomatoes and spice, but there are foods I haven't tried and I really don't know what would happen if I did. A family reunion is not the time to try new foods. So by Dan making my plate, I never even got a look at the food. I also took my own meat, which ensured that it would not be full of histamines or any spices. So over all I think it was a successful day. This is big stuff to me as I spend most of my time at home.

I did get a few questions about my illness, which I actually don't mind. If someone shows an interest, that means they must care. If someone doesn't show any interest, that probably means they don't want to put you on the spot and make you feel interrogated and that is okay too.

I have found you only have a few minutes to answer these types of questions before someone gets foggy- eyed and you lose their interest. How in the world do you explain all of this in just a few minutes? Also, how do you do it without using words that sound like you are just repeating a medical journal?

Well I try to wrap it up in a nice pretty package that looks a little like...

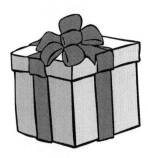 "I have a mast cell disorder. Mast cells are the cells that control your allergy responses. My allergy cells will fire over common things like foods, chemicals and stress. Mine really get upset over salicylates, which are a natural chemical found in all plants. So I have big issues with foods that are plants and products made from plants. Also my mast cells can fire at will, meaning they can get "angry" for no reason."

Short and sweet and to the point without a bunch of medical jargon!

So after these experiences, how does a person not become afraid of everything? I don't know - I am still working on that. Honestly, I am afraid of just about everything, but I can't live life being afraid to move. I guess the bottom line is ...you can't let your fear be bigger than your desire to live. Some days I am better at this than others.

I thought I would share some of those "glamour" shots I mentioned.

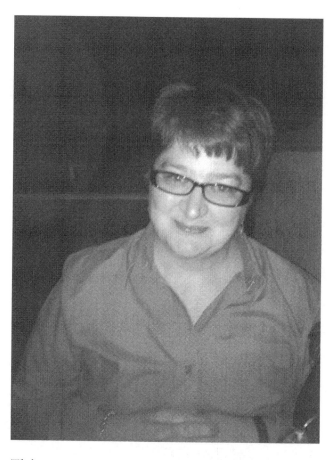

This was me at the beginning of my illness.

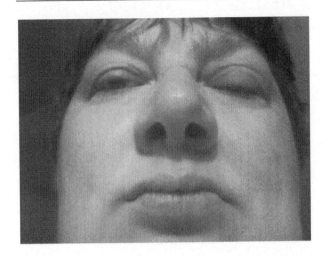

This was the result of an environmental trigger.

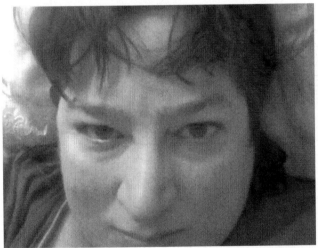

I am convinced that a new appliance caused this.

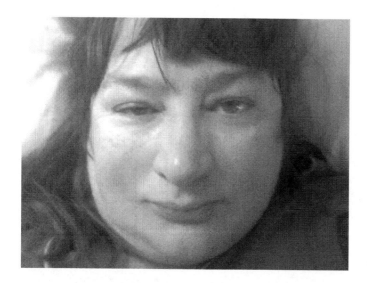

No clue what caused these! It is a mixed bag of crazy!

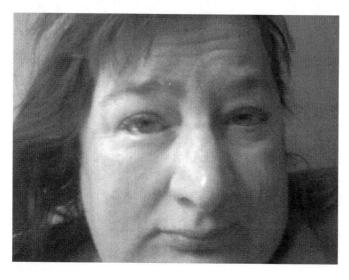

Got to love the hair here!

Chapter 25: Support and Hobbies

"Life is not a solo act. It's a huge collaboration, and we all need to assemble around us the people who care about us and support us in times of strife."

Tim Gunn

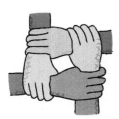 Living with a chronic illness is tough. You need to talk through things, you need answers to questions. Most people who find out they have a chronic illness will join a local support group that meets weekly. But what do you do when there is not a local support group? What do you do when your illness is rare? Thankfully, there is the internet, the amazing conduit to connect you with people all over the world. There is no local mast cell disorder group, but I have my computer to connect with many like me! I have met so many amazing people on the mast cell forums and groups. I met my friend Lori Z. in a forum. She gets me, we have talked for hours on the phone, she has helped me and hopefully I have helped her. She has helped me face things I would not want to face on my own. Thanks, dear friend, I haven't met you in person, but you are still very important to me. I hope we get to meet someday!

Staying busy is also helpful. It is not good to just sit around and think about all the problems we have. That takes a lot of time because, let's face it, we have a lot of problems! I have developed a few new hobbies. I enjoy things that I never took the time to think about before I was sick. Our hobbies may have to change. It is not important what you do, but that you do. Hobbies keep your mind focused, and keep you busy. They also give you something to look forward to.

One of my new hobbies I have taken up keeps me busy and spreads awareness to friends and families of mast cell patients. I have started an Open Face Book Group. My Crazy Life With a Mast Cell Disorder...pretty easy name to remember. It is the only OPEN mast cell group that I am aware of. If you are not comfortable talking about your illness in an open group, if you are trying to keep your illness under wraps, which is perfectly understandable, this would not be the group for you. (Although we do have some members who created a second Facebook account just for health issues - this works.) Some of us don't have a job left or we want to share with our friends and family the crazy things that we go through dealing with this illness. This is the perfect springboard to do that. What better way to learn about this disease than from reading first-hand experiences? I am happy to say we even have a doctor or two who have joined the group to learn!

We share our problems - our ups and downs. We help with questions, with the understanding that we are not doctors, but patients. For the past few years I have been collecting information that is valuable for the members. I post things under 'files' so that people can find the information in the future. It is open for everyone to post things that are important to them. It really is a group effort.

Another hobby includes growing gourds. Now this sounds ridiculous. But they grow so fast that you can see the growth from day to day. I intend to dry the gourds out and make them into bird houses and paint them next year! I have always enjoyed painting so this is a perfect hobby for me. It is a little slower than the painting I used to do but that is okay, because I enjoy it. It is good for me to have enjoyment and take a break from thinking about my crazy life with a mast cell disorder!

Being chronically ill can take a toll on all of your relationships, even the friends and family who stand by you. It is important to show your appreciation for them. A thank you is appreciated by everyone. Don't ever take these people for granted - it is hard work dealing with us sickies. Try to remember they have made a decision to stand by you. Don't ever make them question that decision.

At times, it has been very hard for me to concentrate on too much other than my illness. I am sure I sound like a broken record sometimes. I am trying with all of my might to fight and get well. There is a lot going on physically and emotionally. It is hard emotionally, not be in control of my own body. So people - bear with me when I tell you for the 100th time that I'm triggering and I don't know what is causing it. This is my life I'm battling for...I am on a mission to figure it out. I want to be well again. I want to be the person you remember.

I want to make sure my family knows how grateful I am for their support. My husband has been amazing. We have had stress after stress come at us. Not only illness but loss of jobs, kid's health issues, parent's health issues - you know, all the stuff life throws at you. We have had a lot thrown at us in a span of just a few years. It is very hard to balance it all and remember that we are a team and that we are on the same team. Many couples don't make it through things like this. I have personally spoken to people who have lost relationships due to this illness.

I am thankful for my husband loving me in good times and bad times. Thank you, Dan, for loving me in action. I remember Pastor Grant would always tell us "love is an action, not a feeling." I understand that now...by watching you. Thank you Pastor Grant for teaching us that.

Girls - my sweet, sweet girls. I have seen the frustration in your eyes. Believe me when I say "I understand". You have had your worlds turned upside down, especially you, Bethany. Thank you, Bethany, for all the hours that you sat with me so I wouldn't be alone. Thank you for accepting my limitations with a "that's okay", even when I knew it wasn't okay. Thank you for reminding me of my limitations when I suddenly forget them! I am sorry for all the changes that you all have had to make in your lives. I do appreciate the efforts you all put forth to keep me healthy. When you move out, you can have all the smelly things you want, but I won't visit...and don't wear it when you visit me!

I also want to make a special mention of the friend that has been with me through all of this – Connie. I want to make it clear that I deeply appreciate the friendship we have. I know that we don't see each other often, but we make up for it when we do get together. Some people you just connect with and it doesn't matter how long it is between visits. It is as if you were always around. Thank you for your understanding and your patience. Thank you for sticking by me and never walking away. Thank you for showing me what true friendship looks like.

You never have to wonder if you are making a difference, because you are. I am sorry if I ever made you feel less important than my "closer" friends. Also, I apologize that when we go out to eat we can only go to the same places over and over. Thank you for putting up with that! Maybe someday we can take a fabulous vacation together again. Life happens and you see who is still around. Thanks for still being around!

Future gourd birdhouse!

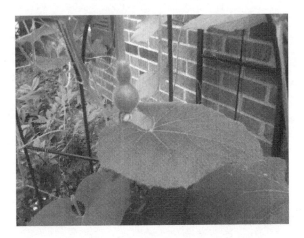

I named this one GourDon, this was my first gourd!

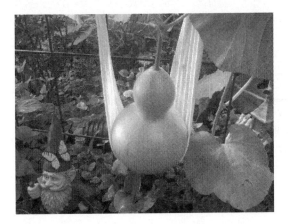

GourDon is so big he needs a sling for the support!

Chapter 26: New Friends

"One of the most beautiful qualities of true friendship is to understand and to be understood."

Lucius Seneca

An amazing thing happened this year with the open group. A friend messaged me and told me he had a friend who just announced she had a mast cell disorder. He is a friend of mine on Facebook. He sees my postings in the group! I was floored! Really?! Where are they, what's their name, is it a guy or gal? I had a million questions. He got permission from her and gave me her name- Janette. It turns out that she lives in the same town. How amazing is that? What is the probability of that? We messaged each other, talked on the phone and finally met in person. By the time we met, it felt like we had known each other for years.

Just having one person who understands what you are going through makes you feel less alone. She just recently got her diagnosis and is not stabilized yet. I tell her she is a "hot mess" because she is! But slowly she is figuring it all out and what is triggering her.

Her most recent discovery is mold in her house. She removed everything you could think that would cause problems - candles, scents, plug-ins, essential oils and carpet. I really do think I was a big pain to her during this process. I would call and ask "have you removed those candles or oils yet?" She would respond, "well not yet, but I don't think that's it". I would repeat the same thing every day. "You need to remove any possible triggers!!" Sorry for being a pain Janette, and a broken record. There is a fine line here between being a nag and a good friend. I was both, but remember I was just concerned for you!

Due to our circumstances with our house, I suggested that she have her air tested for V.O.C.s, mold and formaldehyde. As I said before, we waited two years, which was a mistake; we should have done all of the tests as soon as I got sick. I recommend testing for things in your home right away. Don't make the same mistake we did! We tested for mold, and then waited two years to test for radon, V.O.C.s and formaldehyde. We waited two years...how crazy is that? Think of the time and heartache we could have saved had we just tested everything that first year!

Anyway, they did find high amounts of mold in Janette's house. They are in the process of remediating that. Some friends of theirs loaned them a fancy camper to stay in during the remediation process. You don't want to stay in the house while the problem is being fixed. Hopefully, when their problem is fixed she will see improvements with her health.

She has been a good friend and I hope I have been more of a friend than a pain in the rear. If ever you need a friend, it is when you are at your worst. People will always be around during the highlights of your life, but the dark days are a time people tend to drift off.

I have always gotten fulfillment out of helping people and I have got to help her on a few occasions. On one of those occasions I helped her with her first Epi shot. She was in anaphylaxis and freaking out. I was trying to keep her calm. However, she was not cooperating. I had to take the mean friend approach and tell her "SIT DOWN! I will not chase you around the house with an Epi Pen!" Which may have freaked her out even more, I don't know, but I was there to help and you can't EPi someone while they are running in all different directions! We laugh about it now, so it must not have hurt our friendship too much. I have had the privilege of taking her to the ER and holding her hand and letting her know everything will be okay.

Even though I am stable today, I have no doubt that I will need a friend to take me to an appointment or to the ER someday. It is reassuring to know she is there and willing to help me.

It is funny how things work out. Turns out that our children went to the same school, her son is the same age as Bethany. Apparently, they visited the library where I worked quite often. I think our paths have actually crossed many times and yet it wasn't the right time to meet.

If ever I needed a friend who could understand, it is now. So I am extremely thankful that we met, not too happy about the circumstances, but happy anyway.

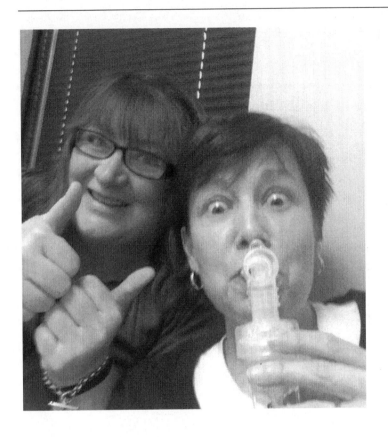

"Walking with a friend in the dark is better than walking alone in the light."

Helen Keller

Chapter 27: Trial and Error and Error

"To make no mistakes is not in the power of man; but from their errors and mistakes the wise and good learn wisdom for the future."

Plutarch

 I have had bad luck with personal products! It took me over 2 years to figure out which shampoo I can actually use. So I am going to share my trial and errors with you. Remember we are all different so what works for me may not work for you.

After dealing with this I can tell you it is much easier to take everything away that could possibly be a problem and then add it back in later. Over the long run it does take less time than removing one item at a time. My motto is to pretend like you live in the 1800's - get rid of foods and products that have unhealthy chemicals in them. If you can't say it, don't eat it or use it! There are suitable substitutes available; you just need to know where to find them. For many months I brushed my teeth, washed my hair and cleaned with just baking soda! It can be done. It makes it very obvious which items are triggers when you go to add something back a month or two later.

Now, being salicylate sensitive adds an element of surprise to actually finding products to use. You go all natural to remove the chemicals, but going all natural means more salicylates, which are just natural chemicals. So, essentially, I have to pick my poison. As I said before, I used baking soda for many things until I felt I was strong enough to try products again. For me it has to be the perfect balance of no salicylates and just a few chemicals.

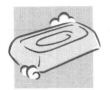

The two hardest products for me to find and use are soap and shampoo. I am letting my hair grow out so the longer it gets the more I feel like I need to wash it. When my hair was super short, it was much easier to take care of but my face is so round that I feel I look better with hair framing my face. Also, the smell in the beauty shop is still a no go for me. I can't possibly deal with that every month.

So I have used lots of salicylate free product lists to find the shampoos, soaps, lotions and make up. (Makeup can be a big trigger, so don't overlook that.) Even though something has been on the list, there were some ingredients that I just could not tolerate. All these products are in my kid's linen closet. I think they have enough to last a few years. When I would go shopping for them, I would buy 3 or 4 different ones at a time just hoping one would work and to save another trip to the store. So after buying and trying 87 shampoos, 35 soaps, several lotions and two kinds of makeup, this is what I found!

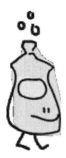

I use the Free and Clear Shampoo that is made by the company that makes the Vanicream. I can also use their hair conditioner. I also use their bar soap- Vanicream Cleansing Bar. You can purchase these products at Wal- Greens, CVS and online. I called the company and they sent me samples of various products including sunscreen, which I haven't been brave enough to try yet!

You can see the products available online here:

http://www.psico.com/

I will sometimes switch out the Vanicream soap for the Aldi brand baby cleanser; it has a nice scent and doesn't seem to bother me. I use this as a bubble bath as well.

Honestly, I try not to use lotion often, if it is not necessary. In the winter it is unavoidable. I do well with the Vanicream Light Lotion, Vanicream Moisturizing Skin Cream or Lubriderm Unscented.

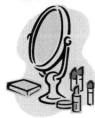

For Makeup and toothpaste I use the Cleure brand. It is found online only. They are gluten-free and hypoallergenic products that are free of parabens, fragrance, and salicylates.

You can see the products available online here:

http://www.cleure.com/

For deodorant I use the Crystal Deodorant found on the Cleure sight or at Walgreens. I have found it online cheaper, but it lasts a long time and I found it just as convenient to purchase on sale at Walgreens. I don't know how the Crystal deodorant actually works, but it does. I will chalk it up to magic! It does not have any harmful chemicals in it. I would love for all my girls to switch to it because it seems so much safer.

For personal products such as Feminine Pads I have found the brand U does not contain Aloe. Aloe is a salicylate, so, for me, many products are problematic. I don't use tampons because let's face it - if I could react to simply being around products, I might react to tampons. This works for me, but I know many women prefer tampons. If this is the case, you might look into some that are all natural and chemical free. I have read some women prefer the Diva Cup and do well with it. It is a silicone cup that is worn internally. I don't think I do great with silicone, so I haven't tried it.

I have found that the Pampers Brand "Baby Fresh" baby wipes are salicylate free. I tried to make my own for a while, but that was not convenient. Wipes you make yourself probably would contain fewer chemicals.

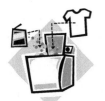 For laundry I use All Free and Clear. I have never had any problem with this so I stick with it.

I do NOT use fabric softener as I think fabric softener is my kryptonite! It is full of chemicals, fragrance and salicylates. I use vinegar in place of fabric softener!

For hand soap I have found that I can use the Wal-Mart clear Equate brand. I have no idea why. I'm pretty sure I found it on a salicylate free list. It is NOT antibacterial. Using antibacterial hand soap is not a good idea because of the chemicals used in it.

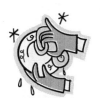 For dish soap I can use small amounts of the green Palmolive.

For the dishwasher we use simple Cascade powder. Those little pod things are so stinky, I can tastes them on the dishes after washing with them. A few ounces of vinegar works wonders as a rinse agent! Shiny dishes every time! Now for a secret...I still have to rely on others to put the dishwashing powder and the vinegar in the dishwasher. I have not found a cleaner that doesn't bother me. So, to this day, I have to go find someone or wait until someone is home to put the soap in and turn it on...So Crazy!

On an even more personal note I can tolerate the Magnum condoms.

I want to mention again about the Epsom Salt bath soaks. Epsom Salt is great for removing toxins from the body. They help with the processing of salicylates. Again...magic, that is all I can come up with! The soaks are also great for sore muscles. I usually soak no longer than 20 minutes; I have read that you reabsorb the toxins that the salt pulls out after about 20 minutes. I started with ¼ cup and slowly worked my way up to 2 cups. You don't want to use more than 2 cups because it is a laxative and it can work as a laxative by absorbing. I found this out when I accidently dropped the whole bag in the water...trust me - it can work as a laxative that way!

If I didn't take the soaks I got pretty sick and even grew fever blisters. Knowing the science behind how they work and growing fever blisters when I didn't take the soaks made it clear to me that I wasn't processing or removing something correctly and the soaks helped with this process. So for a few years I found it beneficial to do a soak every night, except after a big trigger, when I felt a negative reaction. So my advice would be to listen to your body. If you try the Epsom salt soaks, go slowly.

I have been stabilized for about two and half years by taking mast cell stabilizers and the antihistamines. Oh... and let's not leave out that wonderful Singulair!

Although stable, I constantly have to control my environment and my diet. By stable, I mean I am not having out-of-control triggering to foods or my environment. For me, triggering leads to symptoms and symptoms lead to anaphylaxis. Strangely, some days are better than others. I consider it a good week when I have more better days than bad days. I wish I could, for just a moment, not have to think about it. I wish I did not have to calculate every aspect of everything; number of people in the building, amount of fragrance around me at any given time, chemicals used outdoor and indoors, ingredients in foods and medications. I constantly have to be on top of things. That in itself is tiring. Most of the time it is much easier to just stay home than try to go somewhere. I can tell you, I have learned from past experience that I cannot ever, under any circumstances, walk into the left door at Meijer. The chemicals they use in the bathrooms as you walk in are so strong I can smell them from the parking lot. So what does one do when they have to potty at this store? Leave or find the employee bathroom. It is not as deodorized as much as the other bathrooms. There is certainly a learning curve!

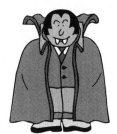 There have been many evenings I had to wear a mask in bed watching t.v. in the clean room because Dan had Mexican or Italian food and it is loaded with garlic - I am like a vampire in this situation too. I may as well break down and make a cape so everyone knows – plus, it would help with the sun burning my flesh!

Your spouse, this is another thing to think about, and this is not in your control. What did they eat for lunch? How will that affect you this evening? Where did they go? What were they exposed to?

At my sickest, I would react to his clothes he wore to church because the church building had a water leak, and although mold was not visible, I can assure you it is there somewhere. It's most likely not at dangerous levels for most people, but it's dangerous to me. Mold is found in every building. I have the same issue with our local Walmart. I still CANNOT go into that store since it leaked. So yes, my mind is constantly trying to calculate risks. I can usually tell what my husband had for lunch after he walks in. I can tell if he had his car washed, not by looking at it but by smelling it. Should I ride in it after he washed it? I don't know. I'm still trying to figure that out. I don't wash my car unless it really, really needs it.

Thankfully, we have the internet because I no longer do fun shopping in stores or the mall. Why risk my life to look at the latest fashion trend. Where would I wear the latest fashions anyway? Also, once I do find something I just love, I have to wash it, like 75 times, to get the formaldehyde and chemicals out of it. It is so much easier for me just stay home and to wear my old favorite shirt. My favorite one is getting pretty bad...my daughter told me the other day I needed some new clothes because my shirt has holes in it. I told her I didn't need new clothes, I just needed a new favorite shirt!

Chapter 28: Crazy Observations

"There are three kinds of men. The one that learns by reading. The few who learn by observation. The rest of them have to pee on the electric fence for themselves."

Will Rogers

I have made several observations over the past few years, things that others may or may not have noticed. Things that my mean something scientific or not! I thought I would share some of these things.

-Before I was put on mast cell stabilizers, any wound I had would heal super-fast, like a super hero! One day while outside I cut my arm and by the next day, it was scabbed and half way healed in a mere 24 hours! Stabilizers calmed down the mast cells, now they are not so active, healing takes longer.

-After a big trigger I will be covered with those little red dots, petechiae. I am guessing this is due to the release of heparin during a reaction.

-A can/bottle of real Coke seems to stabilize me a bit. I have read about caffeine helping to stabilize, so I am 99.9% sure that it's the caffeine in the Coke helping. A Coke is a moderate salicylate and is the only other liquid other than distilled water that I can consume. It also helps with an upset stomach. For obvious reasons I try to drink only one a day. Coke from a fountain contains preservatives, I never drink those.

-I have only recently been able to add a Vitamin C and a Vitamin D into my diet. The funny thing is I can't take them at the same time. This does not work; I have tried it time and time again. Nope- instant diarrhea.

-Seems like I don't have control over my weight. Whether I eat a little or a lot, the weight does not change. I did gain weight when I started on mast cell stabilizers. It is there - it is not going anywhere. At least not going anywhere includes not going up!

-My hair and nails seem to grow at a really fast pace.

-I have not had an infection or illness since I have had a mast cell issue. Like the wound, I think my mast cells attack everything.

-Seemingly little things like hemorrhoids can turn into very BIG deals. The mast cells contribute to inflammation, the inflammation contributes to the problem, the problem makes the mast cells mad, which in turn makes you trigger. This contributes to the original problem. It's a vicious cycle.

-New appliances make me swell - weird and random.

-Every item that touches your skin can leave dermagraphism marks.

-Concentrating on watching a two-hour movie is something I really have to work at.

-Triggering can cause unusual bleeding; again, I believe this is a heparin issue.

-Some days I can eat something, and other days I can't. For some things there is no rhyme or reason, even taking into account that histamines and salicylates stack.

-Clothes seem to be an issue for me - if they are new they contain chemicals, dyes etc. If they are old, they most likely contain fabric softeners. Fabric softeners are so hard to get out. I have washed clothes 150 times in vinegar and baking soda only to have little or no effect on the smell. I have found that soaking clothes in vinegar water for 24 hours does do a good job; however some chemicals just won't wash out.

-Cloudy days seem to be worse for me because of the clouds holding down the exhaust from cars and trains.

-Thrift stores are very hard for me to shop in. I am guessing because of the different detergents, fabric softeners and deodorizers used.

-I do much better with used furniture. However, it has to be new enough that it is not full of odors, but old enough that the chemicals have gassed off.

-When traveling, I take Am Trak . Staying in a private roomette or lower level seems safer for me than flying. I have issues with altitude changes. I even have to medicate on the train when the altitude changes. Plus flying makes me extremely nervous. I avoid being in any space with several people at once; I can't imagine being in an airplane with that many people for several hours. Even though the train takes days instead of hours it is slow and steady for me.

-Strangely, I CANNOT drink milk, but do okay with ice cream or some less aged cheeses. However, I do have to keep these to a minimum because if I over eat dairy products or drink milk I tend to get severe joint pain -- the kind of pain that feels like you have been hit in the knees with a sledgehammer. Very strange!

-Sour cream, which IS high in histamines, makes me itch if it is not brand new! If it is brand new I don't itch but it makes me have the normal high histamine reaction of nausea. If it has been in the refrigerator for several days, and I eat it, I will regret it. This is the only food so far that I know of that makes me itch. It might be because I am not brave enough to try too many other high histamine foods, or maybe it is just because I am stupid enough to try this one. For the record, I usually end up begging someone to remind me the next time that I really, really don't want to eat it!

-When I shop at Sam's club I usually am very drowsy by the time we leave. I am guessing it is due to the many fragrances throughout the huge store along with the fragrances people wear. Even if I am wearing a mask the entire time I usually have to come home and "sleep the stink off". I have stayed home the last few trips so that I don't lose 2 hours shopping and 3 hours sleeping. Also, they use very strong deodorizers in their bathroom. A mast cell patient could get stuck in there for days with diarrhea. The fragrance is so strong it causes diarrhea. Then you have this never ending cycle going on! I avoid their bathrooms if at all possible. I do love their prices on antihistamines though.

- I may have mentioned this, but I have a nose like a dog - I can smell things that no one else can, most of which I have problems with.

-When triggering, I run a low-grade fever. In general my temperature runs pretty low -- around 97.5.

-I have had strange experiences wearing jewelry, like rashes and swelling.

-I have very cold feet. Starting in October I feel as if my toes are frozen until they "thaw out" around May. I think I have poor temperature regulation in my feet.

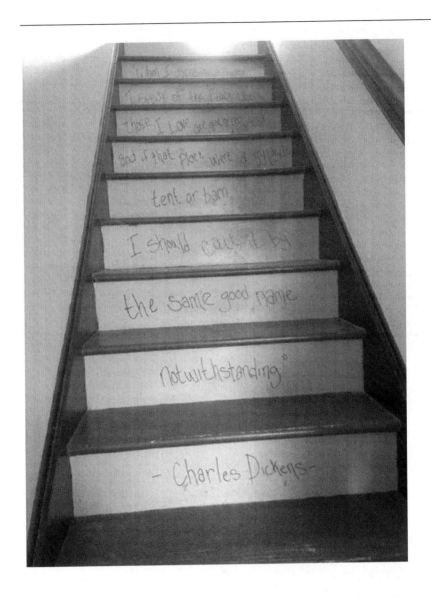

Chapter 29: Foretelling

Remember the foretelling quote?

"When I speak of home, I speak of the place where those I love are gathered together; and if that place were a gypsy's tent, or a barn, I should call it by the same good name notwithstanding."

Charles Dickens

One day I was walking up the stairs and I read that quote from Charles Dickens. It hit me, I had read that quote a million times walking up the stairs, but this time I understood its meaning. I had lived this quote -- whether you are sleeping in a S.U.V., tent, motel or mini-barn, if you have your family with you, you are home!

Why didn't I paint a quote about winning the lottery or having perfect health? It is almost as if I was supposed to learn a life lesson here!

Chapter 30: A Spouse's Perspective

"If you can't handle me at my worst, you don't deserve me at my best."

Marilyn Monroe

I'm Dan, Pam's husband. I wanted to write a few words about my experience with her mast cell disorder over the last 3 years from the spouse's perspective. She has talked to many people in the support groups who have told her that their spouse has a hard time understanding and accepting that they have a chronic illness when there are few outward symptoms. Some spouses go so far as to not believe them at all and believe they are 'faking' or looking for attention. I want to assure them that this is not true.

My wife enjoyed working, especially the interaction with other adults, both co-workers and customers. She really misses that. Now she spends most days alone, interacting with no one. She also enjoyed eating a wide variety of food, as do I. Now she eats the same foods over and over and the only variety of foods I get is when I eat out, and she can't do that often. In addition, she enjoyed going to church and social functions, as well as shopping anywhere she pleased. Now she rarely attends any functions and I do most of the shopping. If you're going to make up an illness, why would you make up one that requires you to give up things you love and creates financial and emotional hardship for your family? That's just stupid. Your spouse needs you to believe and support them. So do that.

Let me assure you that this chronic illness is costing your spouse more than it's costing you. I've witnessed the fear and panic in her eyes as she starts to go into anaphylaxis.

I've witnessed first-hand her taking a cocktail of anti-histamines and H2 blockers in a desperate attempt to avoid using her EPI pen and a trip to the ER. I've witnessed her frustration at the ER or Immediate Care Center with doctors and nurses who've never heard of mast cell disorders or, worse yet, dismiss her symptoms as a panic attack. Sometimes, there's not much you can actually do or say to make things better other than be there with them. So be there.

This is what the "for better or for worse, for richer, for poorer, in sickness and in health" part of your wedding vows was all about. I believe this is one of the reasons that God created the institution of marriage. Anyone will stay with you when you're healthy and wealthy and 'better'. What He desired—and we all need—is someone who will stay with us when we're sick and poor and 'worse'. And you know what? The time may be coming when you'll be on the receiving end of that vow. You will want and need that love and loyalty in return when you're 'worse'. God knows we all need this—he created us, after all. I believe this is God's call on my life right now. God knew that Pam would need someone to be with her, to look after her, to provide for her during this time in her life. I also believe he will hold me responsible if I don't fulfill this calling to the best of my ability.

This calling—like all God's callings—may cost you something. It can create financial hardship with the loss of income coupled with increased medical expenses. Remember, you can't blame your spouse for this. This is not a choice he or she made. Blaming creates anger and anger creates problems. This calling can create emotional hardship as you watch your spouse react to triggers and you feel helpless to do anything but rub their back and stay close, and maybe prepare to go to the hospital. It may also mean you can no longer do things or go places you both used to enjoy. However, you can find new things to do together that you find fulfilling. As long as you're together, that's what's important. So be together.

It may also cost you time and labor. We've ripped up all the carpeting in our house. This isn't a bad idea, anyway. Carpet is filthy. I'm always surprised by what I find when I take out carpet and pad. Of course, there is lots of dust and disintegrated carpet, but I also find flat-out trash. I have found paper, cigarette butts, soda cans, and bowling balls (just kidding). Even for someone who only has allergies, this is a good step. This step, along with better furnace filters and two massive air cleaners, has helped considerably.

The biggest cost for Pam, by far—more than money, eating, working, shopping—has been the cost of friendships. This has actually affected both of us. The husbands of her two closest friends prior to her illness, I considered my closest friends. Pam told you about living in the barn. That was a lot of work. Thankfully, my friend came over to help me after I moved everything from the barn to the garage. I'm glad he helped because he's a better carpenter than I am. He helped me replace the barn window with an actual working window and pick up insulation for the walls. I am very thankful for his help that day. We used to work closely together, mostly related to church business. Sadly, we haven't spoken since his wife started verbally attacking and bullying my wife in a public forum and I asked him to address the issue.

Her closest friend, in my opinion, has issues with not being the center of attention in every situation. I don't know what's wrong with the other one. Something is not right with both of them because mature adults don't act like that. I watched them bully and disrespect Pam — the furthest behavior you would expect from a friend. When they did this, it became awkward for their husbands and I to visit and be friends with the palpable tension and enmity in the air. It is really sad because one of the husbands, in particular, is one of the nicest guys you'll ever meet. I have thought several times how interesting it is that the husbands have been much better friends than their wives. I wonder if that's normal.

I have also thought about how her friends' behavior is being watched by others. People are watching you always — your life is a ministry. What are you teaching? Are you teaching others compassion and understanding or to belittle and hurt those who are already hurting? Are you teaching others to hang on in the bad times or to run when life gets hard?

Let me assure you of one more thing—it gets better. It took several years and even more specialists to finally receive the correct diagnosis. Some of the symptoms of mast cell disorders mimic other conditions. By the time she did receive her diagnosis, Pam had been misdiagnosed with Fibromyalgia, Chronic Fatigue Syndrome and even Lupus. Part of this is because specialists are trained to look for things in their field of specialty so a big part of the solution is finally being referred to the right kind of specialist. Even then, all of the less rare conditions have to be ruled out first, which can take many tests and many months. Now that Pam and her doctor have found the right combination of medications and Pam has identified her triggers and can tell when she's reacting to something sooner and avoid further exposure, she doesn't go 'over the edge', so to speak, nearly as often as she used to. She rarely has to sleep all day anymore and is back to being a wife and not just a sick roommate. So hang on.

Let me conclude by summarizing the above: 1) Your spouse is not faking and has a real disease and needs your support; 2) You made a vow and God expects you to keep it; 3) It may cost you something, but fulfilling your calling is always worth the cost; and 4) It gets better.

Chapter 31: Advice and Wisdom

"The only thing to do with good advice is to pass it on. It is never of any use to oneself."

Oscar Wilde

Here are some great words of wisdom!

Lori Zappella- If I've learned one thing it's that masto giveth, & taketh away. But it gives as good as it gets!

Julia MacDonell

"We are lonesome animals. We spend our life trying to be less lonesome. One of our ancient methods is to tell a story, begging the listener to say - and to feel - Yes, that's the way it is, or at least that's the way I feel it. You're not as alone as you thought."- John Steinbeck

Cary Campanella –"Never leave the house immediately after eating!"

Carrie Bourgo-"How about the disadvantages and advantages to having to wear a mask due to fragrances?!? Like... I can't eat in public (helps with diet control!?!) buuuut burps are trapped in there and it's disgusting ... Hahaha ...Oh and no one can read your lips or hear you if you talk too quietly - which can be ok sometimes if you are muttering angry things but bad when you have to yell at your 4 year old who's took off down the grocery store isle...but advantage is that you can still breathe!"

Terri M.-"I also have learned that a simple trip to the doctor can be very stressful because the thought of trying to explain what masto is or being told " it's nothing " can easily change your mind about going. But you need to go. Not only for your health but piece of mind as well."

Daryl Neal- "Breakthrough!! After 8 years of beating my head against a brick wall...leaving medical clinics and alleged experts in despair...the New Zealand Medical District Health Board is funding a one month Monitored Low Histamine Diet trial for me in Auckland. Yahoo, never give up."

Lori Tedesco Brown- "I tell our friends that I have to handle my husband like an egg out of the carton.

Having Mastocytosis is like being an Egg....I look pretty normal, and I'm hard to peg.

I might be off balance and try to roll on my own....Just keep me nearby with speed dial on your phone.

Don't drop me in hot water, I'll get poached and such...I don't handle temperature changes much.

Try not to scramble me with sausage and cheese....I'll overreact from too many histamines.

Yep, whether I'm over-easy, speckled, hard-boiled, or a different color of shell....We're all in this together dealing with this crazy Mast cell.

P.S....Don't leave me in the sun, I'll sweat and crack...Keep me calm, cool and loved, and I'll love you right back!"

"Masto actually improved my relationship with my husband...he listens to what he's told, tries to eat right, is on anxiety meds alongside his antihistamines and really enjoyed getting a pill organizer in his Easter basket this year!"

Celeste Thomason- "I'm not contagious and my spots are not the chicken pox!"

Tanja Lakić-"Montelukast helped a lot with breathing issues."

Sarah Johnson-"Everyone's always talking about premedicating before surgery which is smart and life-saving, and of course you should do. I learned to Stay Out of the ER (which is just As life-saving sometimes lol) by premedicating before my period hit. And if there was going to be bad weather, plus my period, I made Sure to have as many mast cell stabilizing meds as needed and not to miss any!"

Allie Barnett-"Learn how to not be afraid to tell a doctor, "You're Fired" when you are not getting the treatment and understanding mastocytosis requires."

Julia MacDonell – My favorite quotes-"Keep calm and epi on!"

"Leave me alone - I'm degranulating!"

"If you're nice to me, I'll let you play Connect The Dots!"

Donna Dukes Miller-"Keep looking until you find people who can laugh with you and even at you sometimes. It makes life bearable."

Daryl Neal- "8 years of 2 hour rubbish sleep followed by 2 hours awake leads to CFIDS, it's cognitive dysfunction."

Celeste Thomason- "If we can't laugh at ourselves, what else can we do? Cry I guess and that is okay too!"

Jennifer Dratch- "There's a lot of us who are advanced who still function. I'm in the SM-AHNMD category. I have essential thrombocythemia which is a blood cancer. Due to high platelets I am on baby aspirin, I am doing well. I still work and have pretty good days. I want to make patients aware that it's not the worst thing to advance. I still have a pretty good life going!"

Terri M.-"My favorite or I should say most dreaded question at the doctor's office is 'do you have any allergies?'"

Daryl Neal-"As big as my battle with a mast cell disorder has been, my battle with the medical profession trying to fit me into what they know, has been just as big."

Michelle Starman-"ALL I have to say is if I hear for the 1,000th time but you look so good, and your labs are great how can you be sick, and you even have a great sunburn you must go in the sun a lot UGHHHHHHH!!!!!!!!"

Ellen Myer- "I would want to say to not give up on getting a diagnosis. It has taken most of us an average of about 3 to 4 years, so I have been told. Mine was 4 and was diagnosed as anxiety until then. If you think your children have it too, push! Mine died because I didn't push hard enough, fast enough. It happened right after she was diagnosed but not started on medication for 2 weeks. A moment too late can't be undone. And my other daughter pushed for her child and got her the help she needed. She is 19 and in college- a long ways from the baby in an oxygen tent with diarrhea and screaming in pain. I would want to add just that- don't give up whether or not they get the test results they want the first time."

Janette Egerton-"Every day is a new day. Never give up, never give in."

Alison Babitzke-"Don't stop researching. Both the scientific literature and personal anecdotes from others with chronic illnesses can provide new insights that could prove helpful in your own illness management. I'd also say... In terms of treatment, consider looking into the Paleo Autoimmune Protocol (AIP), which is, in large part, an elimination diet that removes foods that have been scientifically shown to dysregulate the immune system. While the term "autoimmune" may not seem to apply to mast cell disorders, mast cells are a part of the immune system and have the potential to be triggered by certain foods (as many MC patients know!). Currently, I have been following the AIP for seven months. In that time, my life has vastly improved: I have experienced reduction in symptom severity and frequency, been able to taper off several MC meds, and been able to reintroduce several high histamine foods (bacon!). The most thorough resource on the AIP is The Paleo Approach, a book by Sarah Ballantyne, PhD."

Michelle Starman-"POTS is likely to be associated with Mast cell disease. In fact, this was my first diagnosis."

Daryl Neal- Re Mast Cell dysfunction and social media..."If it was easy I guess all of our doctors would know what they are talking about and we'd all be out having fun instead of here seeking answers."

Pat Barker Auston- "Diet matters, natural, fresh, low histamine foods make a big difference but listen to your body. We are all unique!

Karen Wright- "If we all share one little piece of information, maybe we could save others suffering, and blundering in the dark for information as we have had to do."

Tanja Lakić -"Some of the most soothing remedies are love, understanding and compassion from fellow masto sufferers and patience and care from our doctors and families."

Lynda Overgaard- "My couple of thoughts: Why didn't our parents name us; Ana Phil Laxis, or better yet; Em Cass Disease?? You know, some people are bi-lingual, some are bi-racial but how many are biGImotility? *Sorry...couldn't resist :) "

Julia MacDonell-

The Mastocytosis Alphabet:

A - atypical medication use

A - anaphylaxis

A - appetite (loss/gain)

A - antihistamines

B - brain fog

B - bone marrow biopsy

B - bewildered

B - bone pain

B - bathroom

B - "Beauty Marks" (hives and spots!)

C - careful to avoid potential triggers

C - compassion

C - chest pain

C - cutanious

C – canary

D - depression

D - doctors

D - dictionary

D - degranulation

D - The Big D

E - excited *and sad* that I found people like me

E - exercise intolerance

E - Epi-pen

E - every day

E - exasperation

E - exhausting

E - embarrassment

F - fighting for a cure

F - frustrated

F - friends in unexpected places

F - fatigue

F - flushing

F – food: yes? no?

G - goofy behaviors

G - gut rebellion

G - good ideas to share

H - histamine

H - hope

H - hives

H - humility

H - help

H - hypertension

H - headaches

H - humor

H - hot

I - ice cold feet

I - idiopathic

I - itching

I - irritation: both kinds

I - "I don't know"

J - jelly for brains

J - jittery

J - jeopardy

J - joint pain

J - jumpy

J - junction: turning a new corner

K - Ketotifen: my new best friend

K - kindness of strangers

K - klutzy

L - lassitude: on bad days

L - love

L - lethargic

L - learning

L - Leukotrienes

M - Mast Cell Stabilizers!!! yay!!

M - mast cells

M - muscle pain

M - meds

M - malabsorption

N - new experiences

N - neuropathy

N - never-ending

N - nuisance

N - neoplasm

N - night-sweats

N - new normal

O - osteoporosis

O - orphan diseases

O - outcast

P- pain pain and more pain

P - pruritis

P - pathology

P - pressure

P - Prostaglandins

Q - quirky reactions

Q - Quercitin

Q - queasy

Q - questions, questions, QUESTIONS!

R - rash

R - REST!

R - rare

S - swelling

S - systemic

S - syncope

S - support

S - surprises

S - stress

S - strength

S - scary

S - sucks

T - tears of frustration

T - tired

T- tachycardia

T - Tryptase

T - tests, tests, tests

U - uncomfortable

U - unusual

U - Urticaria Pigmentosa

V - vomiting

V - vexing

V - vertigo

V - variety

W - waiting

W - worrying

W - water retention

W - what??

X - x-rays

X - Xanax

Y- yucky: how I feel a lot of the time

Y - yo-yo health

Y - yes: today might be a good day

Z - zaps energy

Z - Zyrtec and Zantac our H1 and H2 blockers

References & Helpful Links

Link to a list of patient recommended doctors who treat mast cell disorders: https://www.facebook.com/notes/my-crazy-life-with-mast-cell-disorder/recommended-doctors/378985405540771

The Mastocytosis Society, Inc.: http://www.tmsforacure.org/welcome.php

My Crazy Life With A Mast Cell Disorder Support Group: https://www.facebook.com/groups/344270359012276/

My rare disease day video: https://www.youtube.com/watch?v=zVhHaTGiG3I

Patient experience with Mastocytosis: http://www.mastocytosis.ca/MSC%20Patient%20Experience%20April2012.pdf

Other diseases to consider or rule out : https://www.facebook.com/notes/my-crazy-life-with-mast-cell-disorder/not-mast-cell-disorder/429771213795523

http://salicylatesensitivity.com/

http://www.tmsforacure.org/documents/ChroniclesSE.pdfhttp://www.ncbi.nlm.nih.gov/pmc/articles/PMC3069946/table/T5/

To purchase masks: http://www.vogmask.com/

To make your own mask: https://www.facebook.com/groups/344270359012276/540935706012406/

To check your drug interactions: http://www.drugs.com/

To check the ingredients in your drugs:
http://pillbox.nlm.nih.gov/pillimage/search.php

To view "files" of My Crazy Life With a Mast Cell
Disorder: https://www.face-
book.com/groups/344270359012276/files/

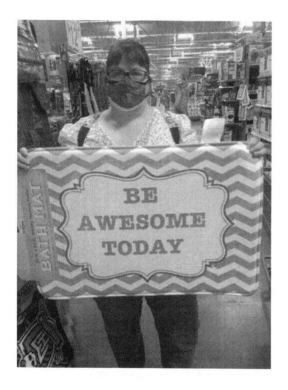

Made in the USA
San Bernardino, CA
08 July 2017